LIVING IN
SYNCHRONY

I0104933

Books by Amy L. Lansky

Impossible Cure
Active Consciousness
Living in Synchrony

Praise for *Impossible Cure*:

"An introduction to homeopathy that stands out from the rest."
—Dr. Joseph Mercola, *Mercola Newsletter*

"The finest general introduction to homeopathy I've yet read."
—Julian Winston, Author: *The Faces of Homeopathy*

"We have never had this kind of response to an introductory book."
—Greg Cooper, Minimum Price Homeopathic Books

Praise for *Active Consciousness*:

"This book is a gift—well written, coherent, purposeful, and clear. I recommend it to all seekers of deeper awareness and consciousness."
—Vatsala Sperling, PhD, Reviewer for *Homeopathy Today*

"This is a delightful book. Well written and intensely packed with interesting information. It made my head spin—in a good way!"
—Dean Radin, Author of *The Conscious Universe* and *Entangled Minds*

"After reading this, you will hold on to your personal power for dear life. You will have a new understanding of the power that lies within the choices we make, and how those create new realities all the time."
—Danut Incrosnatu, *One of 5 spiritual books that will change your perspective of reality*

"Amy Lansky's brilliant attempt to bridge the connection between stilling the mind and influencing reality with our thoughts."
—Jair Robles, *superconsciousness.com*

LIVING IN SYNCHRONY

A GUIDE TO HEALING AND RECLAIMING OUR POWERFUL, NATURAL HUMANITY

Amy L. Lansky, PhD

R.L.Ranch

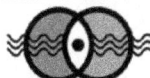

Press

Greenville, South Carolina

Living In Synchrony: A Guide to Healing and Reclaiming Our Powerful, Natural Humanity

Copyright © 2025 by Amy L. Lansky, PhD
www.amylansky.com

Printed and bound in the United States of America. All rights reserved. No part of this book may be reproduced or transmitted in any form or by an electronic or mechanical means, including photocopying, recording, or by an information storage and retrieval system, without permission from the Publisher—except in the case of brief quotations embodied in reviews and academic papers.

No AI training. Without in any way limiting the author's and publisher's exclusive rights under copyright, any use of this publication to train generative artificial intelligence (AI) technologies to generate text is expressly prohibited. The author reserves all rights to license uses of this work for generative AI training and development of machine learning language models.

For more information, please contact: R.L.Ranch Press. E-mail: info@rlranchpress.com. Visit *www.amylansky.com* to find out more about the content of this book and ordering information.

Although the author and publisher have exhaustively researched all sources to ensure the accuracy and completeness of information contained in this book, we assume no responsibility for errors, inaccuracies, omissions, or any inconsistency herein. Any slights of people, places, or organizations are unintentional.

Special note to reader. Although this book describes several methods for healing, self-development, and empowerment, it is not meant to give specific recommendations of psychological, medical, or other advice. Nor does it make any warranties or guarantees of any sort that any information in this book or on *www.amylansky.com* will produce any particular physical, emotional, or other result.

ISBN: 978-17320879-27 (ISBN-10: 1-7320879-2X)

Cover art by Amy Lansky
Cover design by Steve Rubin
Interior design by Steve Rubin, based on a design by Melanie Haage
Illustrations and figures by Max Rubin and Steve Rubin
Author photo by Jennifer Dungan

For the intrepid ones,
who follow their own truth and wisdom,
rather than the safety of the crowd

TABLE OF CONTENTS

Foreword   ix

Acknowledgments   xii

Introduction   1

PART I.   Change Your Vibration, Change Your Life

Chapter 1.   It's All About Vibration   9
The Origin of Our Habitual State; What is Physical and Emotional Disease?

Chapter 2.   What Is "Living in Synchrony"?   17

Chapter 3.   Open and Expand Your View   22
Will You Consider Age Old Wisdom or Stick to Modern Convenience?; The Imperative of Frontier Science; A Revolution Is Coming; What You Will Find in This Book; It Goes Beyond Personal Healing

PART II.   What's *Really* Going On?

Chapter 4.   The Box   37
Stop the Chatter and Look Within; Beyond the Box

Chapter 5.   Who Are We? What Are We?   46
The Energy Body Architecture; The Etheric Body; The Central Channel

Chapter 6.   Beyond the Physical and Etheric   54
The Astral Body; Death and Out-of-Body Experiences (OBEs); A Higher Dimensional World; Sleep, Lucid Dreams, and OBEs

Chapter 7.   An Astral Journey, Part I   67

Chapter 8.   I Think *and* I Am   71
The Mental Body; The Role of the Mental Body; The Causal Body

Chapter 9. Opening the Door of Creation   80
  The Ha Ritual

Chapter 10. An Astral Journey, Part II   87

Chapter 11. A Greater Cosmology   91
  Visualizing What We Are; Animals, Elementals, and Divas; Oversouls and
  Angelic Beings

Chapter 12. The Purpose of Life   97

PART III.   Find Your Path to Healing

Chapter 13. Healing From the Outside In   105
  My Own Healing Journey; The Levels of Our Being; Each Level Has Inherent
  Healing Power

Chapter 14. We Are Physical Beings   114
  Signs and Cautions for the Physical Realm; Physically-Based Therapies;
  Approaches That Add Something to or Subtract Something from Your Body:
  Conventional Medicine (surgery and drugs); Diet and Supplementation; Herbal
  Medicine; Detoxification; Approaches that Externally Manipulate Your Body
  and Its Organs and Systems: Exercise and Physical Therapy; Posture
  Therapies; Movement Therapies and Massage; Chiropractic and Osteopathy

Chapter 15. We Are Beings Governed by Energy and Vibration   148
  Signs and Cautions for the Etheric Realm; Etherically-Based Therapies;
  Approaches That Access the Etheric Body Through Physical Interventions That
  Insert Something Into the Body: Homeopathy; Traditional Chinese Medicine
  (TCM); Approaches That Access the Etheric Body Only Through Touch,
  Movement, or External Energies: Hands-on Healing: Energy Exercises; Sound
  Therapies; Healing with Crystals and Geometry; Muscle Testing (Applied
  Kinesiology)

Chapter 16. We Are Emotional Psychic Beings   180
  Signs and Cautions for the Astral Realm; Astral Body Recap; Astrally-Based
  Therapies; Approaches That Work By Simply Acknowledging the Powerful
  Role of the Astral Body: The Work of Dr. John Sarno and TMS;
  Communicate with the Astral Body: Psychotherapy; Hypnotherapy; Journaling,
  Meditation, Automatic Writing, and Divination Methods; Mirror Work, Self-
  compassion, Self-love; The Sedona Method; Core Transformation; Family

Constellation Therapy; Connect with the Astral Body Via the Physical Body: EFT (Emotional Freedom Technique) and TFT (Thought Field Therapy); EMDR (Eye Movement Desensitization and Reprocessing); TRE (Trauma Release Exercises); Breathwork, Sweat Lodges, Ecstatic Dance, Sound, and Plant Medicine; Shamanism

Chapter 17. We Are Willful, Thinking, Meaning-full Beings   218
Untangle Your Perception of Your Higher Bodies; Meaning; The Power Of Will; Disease Within the Mental Body; Signs and Cautions for the Mental Realm; Mentally-Based Therapies; Look Back; In the Present Moment, Look More Deeply Within and Without; Look Forward

Chapter 18. We Are Creators   237
The Law of Attraction; Manifestation/Creation Methods Based on the Law of Attraction; Problems in the Causal Body; Signs and Cautions for the Causal Realm; Causally-Based Therapies; The Basic Manifestation/Creation Process; Embellishments on the Theme: Huna; The Teachings of Neville Goddard; The Teachings of Joe Dispenza; Clearing Obstacles: The Teachings of Abraham Hicks; The Science of Mind; Some More Thoughts on Letting Go

Chapter 19. You Are Not Alone   256
Being Part of a Collective; Collective Healing at the Physical Level; Collective Healing at the Etheric Level; Collective Healing at the Astral Level; Collective Healing at the Mental Level; Collective Healing at the Causal Level

Chapter 20. Ultimately, We Are One   275
Move Forward into Healing

Notes and Resources   282

Bibliography   293

Assorted Websites   298

Selected Index   301

About the Author   304

FOREWORD

Like a "house built on rock," Amy Lansky lays the foundation of her thesis on solid evidence and then creates a dwelling place that is both artistic and practical. She combines the wonderful insights of energy medicine (e.g., homeopathy), deep familiarity with esoteric thought, and a career in computer science. Amy has created a beautiful logical arrangement of her thesis—each part flowing seamlessly and informing the next. The elegance of this organization and the organic flow of her material sweeps the readers along effortlessly, allowing them to appreciate the scenery en route while eagerly anticipating the destination, which is a conclusion reminiscent of the Eight Beatitudes of Jesus and the Eightfold path of the Buddha.

Amy's ability to move from the individual to the collective (families, cultures, nations, religions, governments) affords the reader an eagle's-eye view of the issues under discussion. In one powerful paragraph, early in the book, she says, "Truthfully, these concepts can go way beyond personal healing. They apply to all of the living things on Earth and to the Earth itself. They may even apply to the solar system, galaxy, and universe!"

Her book is also filled with pithy one-liners. For example, in part of her historical review of paradigm shifts she says, "But within each civilization, the wise ones tended to focus on meaning rather than money, on enlightenment rather than entertainment." Later in the book, she says, "If our beliefs can create our reality, then our experienced reality tells us something about our beliefs."

The building stones of Amy Lansky's edifice are insights from Hippocrates, Maimonides, Jung, Steiner, Gurdjieff, Ibrahim Karim, and a host of others. In a wonderful cosmological flip, she replaces the idea that progress consists of the *acquisition of higher levels of the Self* with the notion that progress is really about *shedding our identification with lower levels of the Self*. In my experience, Amy's exegesis of the many levels of the Self—

physical, etheric, astral, mental and causal—is the best I've ever encountered.

Amy also peppers her tome with practical exercises that awaken the energies of all levels of the Self—leading us in a dance between outer teachers and inner guidance. Like a great teacher she tells us what she is *going to teach*, then she *teaches it* and, finally, she synopsizes what she has *just taught*. And when it comes to healing modalities, she doesn't just have a theoretical knowledge of her topic, she has "test-driven" many of them. This book is a manual that shows you how to pop the hood of your incarnational automobile and make the necessary repairs and upgrades.

The function of a real prophet is not to *foretell* the future but to *forestall* it; not to *predict* the future but to *prevent* it. For the prophet is one who sees the present so clearly that she can judge where it's headed. Thus, there are two types of "future"—the *probable* future, if we don't listen to the prophet and change our behavior, and the *possible* future if we do listen and make the changes. The scriptures are filled with false prophets who tell the rulers what the rulers want to hear. And secular history is replete with "court historians" who sing the praises of the current crop of tyrants. I put Amy Lansky into the group of true prophets. She has the courage to call out the tyrannies of the COVID-era.

Like Sarah and Abraham of old, Amy and her husband, Steve, had the courage to set out from the land of the idol-makers and seek freedom. They sought a land flowing with "milk and honey" in place of a swamp drowning in greed and hubris. She is willing to take on not just government bureaucrats, but the pharmaceutical industry and even her old colleagues in Silicon Valley—the AI transhumanists who are attempting to create what I call, "Homo Artificialis." She's not afraid to call out and challenge the hydra-headed corruption that puts power and profit ahead of human health and happiness.

Years ago, I coined the term, "mysticist" to mean a kind of a gnostic intermediary—one who is proficient in both science and spirituality, a cross between a mystic and a scientist. I had people like Teilhard de Chardin in mind—a Jesuit priest and paleoanthropologist as well as mystical soul-seeker. I would put Amy Lansky in that category also. In this magnum opus, she combines real psycho-physiological science with both trenchant data-driven arguments and crystal-clear writing.

Well done, Amy!

Fr. Seán ÓLaoire – Tír na nÓg
Spiritual Director of Companions on the Journey
Author of *Setting God Free*
www.spiritsinspacesuits.com
December 2024

ACKNOWLEDGMENTS

It is said that the expression of gratitude brings more goodness your way. If so, I may have a lot of wonderful things to look forward to! When you think about it, this principle is actually synchronicity in action. Here are some gratitudes that I'd like to share with you.

First of all, I am so grateful for my life and all the teachers and healers that have come into it. Without them, I would never have been able to write this book. Indeed, this book is my way of imparting to you, the reader, what I have learned over my nearly 70 years. In my opinion, the purpose of life is to grow and learn and then share it with others. That has been my goal in writing this and my previous two books, *Impossible Cure* and *Active Consciousness*.

Second, I am grateful for all the twists and turns that have brought me to this point. That especially includes my family: my husband and companion on this incredible life journey, Steve Rubin, and my children and teachers, Izaak and Max. They are the foundation for everything I do. My 44 years with Steve have been my greatest blessing, from our wild and nerdy rock'n'rolling days in Silicon Valley of the 80s, to the discovery of homeopathy that healed our son Max and then delivered all four of us, to our growing involvement in the health freedom community, and ultimately our voyage across America that led us to the American South, a place we have grown to love and embrace. We have seen and learned so much!

Third, I am grateful to all the people who have read and/or given me feedback on versions of this book—both its initial incarnation (Carolyn Scott, Chris Wellens, Palmer Kippola, Denny Brown, Ashmi Pathela, and Steve and Izaak Rubin) and its transformed, final version (Andi Stowe, Allison Durazo, Kathleen Lunn, and Steve Rubin). I am also immensely grateful to Father Seán ÓLaoire, who answered my "cold call" request to write the Forward for *Living in Synchrony* and said yes! Steve and I listened to Seán's homilies throughout our voyage of transition from Silicon Valley to South Carolina (and still listen). His teaching helped to give us courage and confidence. I also want to acknowledge the love and support of so many friends, both old and new. That includes our old friends and family in Silicon Valley and our hometowns in Buffalo and New Jersey, our newer friends in the homeopathy and health freedom worlds, and our newest friends and neighbors in South and North Carolina.

Finally, I want to acknowledge the bravery of those who did not fall under the spell of mass formation during the COVID years and stood up to powerful forces in the media, government, business, and Big Pharma. My prayer is that more and more of us wake up and do not fall into secondary formations brewing on all sides. Be discerning! This will be especially important and difficult as the tsunami of artificial intelligence, media manipulation, genetic engineering, and surveillance grows ever stronger.

Let's hang on, with all our might, to our powerful, natural, humanity!

INTRODUCTION

If the COVID years taught me anything, it's that life can be unpredictable and mysterious. Each day presented a shifting picture of reality: what I could or couldn't do, where I could or couldn't go, and who I could or couldn't believe or depend upon. I learned to reconsider things that I had never really questioned before. What was true and what was false? Was the information repeated by the media correct? Indeed, once trusted sources now came up for question and deeper scrutiny.

Fairly quickly, the predictable lives that most of us led were replaced by a time in which we couldn't plan more than a few days ahead. Life trajectories that I would have considered unbelievable became new futures that lay before me. In the end, my husband Steve and I left our home in the San Francisco Bay Area—a home we had lived in for 38 years and thought we'd live in until we died—and moved to another state across the country, one that we had never been to and knew nothing about. We did this after driving over 17,000 miles around the USA, living in hotels for nearly seven months, and visiting dozens of cities. Our goal: to find a new home, a place where we could feel peaceful and comfortable with both the surroundings and the people.

In many ways, this unexpected experience was a gift. It forced Steve and me to live day to day, trusting in what the universe presented to us. When we first hit the road in mid-2021, we consciously decided to listen to the hints and clues and synchronicities we met up with along the way. Friendly strangers directed us. Hotel mishaps redirected us. We learned to take life more in stride and to trust in what God—the force that creates and underlies our consciously experienced reality, as well as other unseen realities—bestowed upon us. Our search was exhausting and exhilarating at the same time. You might call it *"living in synchrony."*

More about what that phrase means later. But for now, let me tell you a bit more about myself and why you might be interested in what I have to say in this book.

I spent the first part of my working life as a researcher in computer science, with most of my efforts in the field of artificial intelligence (AI), albeit an older form of AI that bears no resemblance to the kind now overtaking human society. I received my doctorate in computer science from Stanford University and worked in Silicon Valley during its first heyday—the 1980s and 1990s, a time of great excitement and optimism. I personally know many people who later became key power players in the tech world, and as a result, I believe I understand much more deeply than most people do about the potential pitfalls and dangers we may soon face as a global civilization.

As fate would have it, however, I left the Silicon Valley rat race in the late 1990s when my younger son became an early victim of the now-mushrooming autism epidemic. Luckily for our family, we discovered the miraculous healing power of homeopathic medicine. Over the next several years, our son made a complete recovery. Eventually, I studied homeopathy and wrote what is still a leading popular introductory text on the subject, *Impossible Cure: The Promise of Homeopathy*. I also became deeply involved in promoting and trying to safeguard patient access to this powerful and unique form of medicine.

After working in the alternative health arena for several years, I decided to branch out further and began an exploration of more esoteric subjects—things like meditation, synchronicity, and manifestation techniques. Eventually, I wrote a second book, *Active Consciousness: Awakening the Power Within,* which weaved all of these subjects together, including their relationship to homeopathy.

Now you are reading my third book, *Living in Synchrony*. It embodies a deepening and broadening of my first two books, and focuses not only on a myriad of alternative treatment possibilities, but also provides guidance in how to explore them. I learned about these modalities in my own quest to heal myself and my family over the years. Most of them address levels of our being that go way beyond our physical bodies and deal with the so-called "energy bodies," parts of us that operate within unseen realms. And despite the fact that we may not see them, they *do* affect our physical bodies in profound ways.

Of course, many people were interested in alternative medicine, the energy bodies, synchronicity, and manifestation techniques long before COVID. But for me and Steve, our experiences during the pandemic made these subjects much more palpable and real; it expanded our understanding of and belief in them. As our time on the road untethered us from our previous lives, we seemed to be directed by invisible forces that guided and helped us. Naturally, we had to deal with day-to-day details too; it wasn't a magical mystery tour. We had to book hotels, find restaurants, and pack and unpack our bags over and over again. And when we did wind up getting COVID on the road, it was homeopathy that made the biggest difference in healing us.

Not surprisingly, this voyage made a lasting impact upon us. What had been intellectual beliefs before became experienced realities. It cemented in our minds the fact that, yes, the world truly *is* mysterious and our bodies and life *do* operate in ways humanity is only beginning to fathom. As Steve and I often said to one another in yet another hotel room in yet another town along the way (and still say to one another!): "Where are we?" "What is going on?" Now we both trust more than ever in the underlying benevolence of our unfolding reality, in the directives we receive along the way, and in the miraculous healing power of alternative approaches to health. Although I completed the first draft of this book in mid-2020, it was our experiences during our voyage across America that clarified the true purpose of *Living in Synchrony* for me.

All of humanity is going through a process of upheaval right now. Most people are coping by trying to return to their "old lives." Many seek comfort in putting up figurative and often literal walls of control in order to provide a sense of security. Such folks may welcome efforts to increasingly regulate and surveille their lives and bodies, because they believe it will create a kind of risk-free living.

Ultimately, however, I believe that such efforts are misguided band-aid solutions. Ominously, they are also usually offered to us by entities that have their own interests at heart—usually financial gain and power. Add to this picture the increasing ubiquity of technology in society and the even more frightening efforts to incorporate technologies *into* our bodies; that is, the move toward *transhumanism*—in essence, the merger of man and machine. *I believe that such developments will soon pose a risk to our lives as free and truly natural human beings, and that they might also disempower our healing abilities in fundamental ways.*

Sadly, one of the key centers of development for these technologies is my alma mater, Stanford University, as well as the greater San Francisco Bay Area that surrounds it. That fact alone contributed to Steve's and my decision to leave our lives there behind. If you believe that transforming into a genetically-engineered cyborg will be to your benefit and convenience, please realize that if your survival depends upon drugs and machinery that could be controlled by others, you have surely enslaved yourself.

When you think about it, the amount of censorship and control over information and personal freedom enacted during the COVID years is reminiscent of the world described in the prophetic book *1984* written by George Orwell back in 1949. Life in China today already looks like a modern version of it, with its social credit system, propaganda machine, and extreme forms of surveillance. But even in the Western world, these sorts of things are being enacted—albeit in more subtle ways. On top of this, with accelerating advances in bioengineering of not only our food but also our bodies, we also seem to be marching toward the world described by writer Aldous Huxley in another prophetic book, *Brave New World*, published in 1932.

It's time to wake up!

Instead of continuing along this path, let's remember some age-old wisdom: *the Earth and our collective humanity have inherent powers all their own.* Things are operating in ways that none of us can see, no one can control, and certainly no one can ever truly understand. In other words, the world is inherently unpredictable and mysterious! As a result, our efforts to artificially control our lives and bodies will likely meet with unforeseen and unfortunate consequences.

Now is the time for us to embrace and protect our complete and natural humanity, our complete and natural Earth. We are self-healing wonders and we live on an inherently self-healing Earth. We just need to get out of the way and foster these natural processes, not forcibly control them.

This book is an effort to help you realize and embrace that truth. You might think of it as a survival manual for the coming times—times in which many of us may require the ability to heal ourselves rather than rely on conventional institutional health structures. This was true of the American pioneers as they traveled across the brutal western frontier, and it has always been true of indigenous people around the world. Today, an increasing number of people are realizing that they, too, are pioneers exploring an unpredictable future. My hope is that this book will help guide you as you embark upon your own journey.

Before you can proceed, however, you need to better understand the nature of your complete being or Self—in particular, how it is comprised of much more than just your physical body. That's why I structured this book in the way that I did. Part I begins by introducing you to some key concepts and, in particular, the critical role of *vibration*. Next, in Part II, I present an expanded view or model of who and what we truly are. This model will then help you to decide which of the healing tools described in Part III have the most potential for you. Put all of this together and you will gain access to new options, new power, and new awareness. So, let's get started!

PART I

CHANGE YOUR VIBRATION, CHANGE YOUR LIFE

"To know that what is impenetrable to us really exists, manifesting itself as the highest wisdom and the most radiant beauty which our dull faculties can comprehend only in their most primitive forms—this knowledge, this feeling, is at the center of all true religiousness. In this sense... I belong in the ranks of devoutly religious men."
–Albert Einstein

CHAPTER 1

>

IT'S ALL ABOUT VIBRATION

When it comes to the reality that we experience each day, it's really all about *vibration*—or frequency, if you prefer. It may seem like the material objects around you are solid and fixed, but physics tells us that at the lowest level of scientifically-proven reality—the quantum level—our universe is a pulsating vibe. Our bodies, the plants around us, the rocks, clouds, and air we breathe, are all, ultimately, complex vibrations—each mineral, plant, and animal playing its own personal tune. And even if we're not consciously aware of the vibrational symphony being played all around us, we *are* affected by it.

Most of us know what it feels like when we are in resonance with someone—the feeling that we are "on the same wavelength." We even use the language of vibration to describe it. And we can certainly sense it when someone "turns us off," even if we don't exactly know why. Many of us can also detect if something isn't quite right as we enter a house where unhappiness prevails. Or we feel a sense of unease when a relative or friend is in trouble, even if we don't consciously know about it. Scientific studies have even demonstrated that when two people are emotionally connected, their bodily readings can literally synchronize, even when they are separated by steel walls or great distances.[1] Perhaps vibrational effects are also why people can be healed in the presence of energetically powerful and gifted individuals.

This phenomenon is not just the result of human imagination, the power of suggestion, or the so-called "placebo effect." In fact, studies that I will describe in Chapter 3 demonstrate that even the behavior of *machines* can be affected when a large group of people is experiencing strong emotions, especially negative ones.[2] We all know that group energy can be "contagious." Well, it's contagious to machines too!

As this book will discuss, vibration also likely characterizes even subtler levels of reality than the quantum level. We may not be able to perceive these realms, or we may actively disbelieve in their existence, but I believe every one of us lives within, interacts with, and is affected by these subtle levels of reality, whether we acknowledge them or not.

So why is vibration so important? If I had to sum up a key message of this book in one sentence it would be:

In order to fundamentally change and improve your health and your life, you must shift to a new state of vibration.

I'll grant you—it's not always easy to do. For one thing, most of us aren't even aware that we're stuck in a state of vibration that's making us ill or unhappy or unsuccessful. And shifting can be difficult because we tend to be *habituated* to our baseline state of being. That is, it feels "normal" to us, even if it's unpleasant physically or emotionally. In fact, it may be all we've known since childhood. Because of this, shifting to a new state of vibration can feel strange or uncomfortable initially. But in order to find the peace and health you desire, it's absolutely imperative that you try.

There is also an important corollary to this vibrational maxim, and it has to do with external alignment with your environment:

To feel happy and healthy in a particular environment, your personal state of vibration must be in alignment with your environment's state of vibration.

As I said in the introduction, one of the major reasons why Steve and I decided to leave California (and Silicon Valley in particular) was that we increasingly felt it was no longer in alignment with who we had become. Over the course of several years, our vibration had changed—and so had the vibration of Silicon Valley itself. These two vibrational states now clashed and we personally no longer felt good there, even though it took us a long time to understand why that was true. Because of this, one of the guiding principles we used when choosing our new homeland was to find a place where we did feel comfortable, at ease, and *at home*. Some people may still flock to Silicon Valley because they *are* in alignment with its new vibration. But it was no longer right for us. Today, I understand more deeply that it was actually all about the phenomenon of vibration.

I believe that many people on Earth are now becoming more aware of, or at least sensitive to, this truth. With shifts and increasing extremes in societal polarities emerging all over the planet, it is no wonder that many folks are feeling increasingly ill at ease. In the United States, for example, the COVID years sparked a remarkable movement in population that is still ongoing. Is something happening on a deeper vibrational level, beyond economics and politics? Is that why more and more people are feeling the urge to move locales just like Steve and I did—in order to find an inner sense of alignment once again?

Some have even suggested that a major bifurcation in vibrational realities is emerging, with Earth reality splitting into two future timelines. If so, which possible future do you want to be a part of? Is a technological and controlled future appealing to you? Or one that is natural, spiritual, and human-centered? Now may truly be the right time for you to make your choice and act. Perhaps that's one reason you are reading this book.

THE ORIGIN OF OUR HABITUAL STATE

Let's get back to personal vibration. Why would anyone develop an unhelpful state of vibration in the first place? It certainly doesn't seem like a good survival strategy. The fact is, however, that it *is* about survival. Usually, some event or family situation fostered this vibe within us when we were children. It was strategically useful and appropriate back then and it helped us to survive. The trouble is, it may not be serving us anymore. Moreover, because we're so used to it, we don't even notice it or recognize its downsides. Unfortunately, such lifelong habitual states are often the root cause of chronic disease and interpersonal dysfunction. Indeed, much has been written, especially recently, about the physical and emotional impacts of childhood trauma.

I'll give you an example from my own experience. I grew up in a family with a powerful and demanding father who could suddenly become violent toward my mentally ill older brother. There were even occasions when I physically stepped in to defend my brother. Although my mother was never around during these episodes, her attention was generally consumed by having to deal with my brother's health and his negative interactions with my father. Eventually, she developed a chronic state of mild depression that rendered her emotionally inaccessible to me.

Put all of this together and you can understand the survival strategy I developed. To garner whatever love, attention, and approval I could get from my father, I tried to be the "perfect" child—the talented and successful one. This had the side benefit of teaching me grit and tenacity. To cope with my mother's absence, I learned to be self-sufficient emotionally. Unfortunately, along with this came a lot of downsides:

perfectionism, anxiety, the feeling that I constantly needed to be on the alert (because of my father's hair-trigger temper), survivor's guilt, the feeling that I needed to fix everything (because of my brother's situation), and feelings of disappointment and abandonment. The truth is, however, that this chronic state of being no longer serves me and is at the root of many of the physical symptoms I've developed as I've aged.

So how can we leave a chronic, habitual state of vibration behind? One thing I've learned over the past few years is that with some effort, it *is* possible to make progress. Sure, we often backslide into our old coping mechanisms, especially in times of stress. But we can become much more aware of it when we do. That's the first step. Awareness. Naming it. Accepting and, in a way, getting into alignment with what's actually going on. Once we are able to catch ourselves, we can then use a variety of tools that help us to break free of negative patterns and develop a new way of being—in other words, to heal. It's not about suppressing or blocking our habitual state. It's about awareness, acceptance, and finally, transcendence.

What Is Physical and Emotional Disease?

Simply stated, disease is an unhealthy state of being; an unpleasant "vibe." Its cause might be physical, emotional, or environmental. A car accident. A virus. The loss of a loved one. It could be some toxic spew from a pesticide or a careless comment from a relative. Usually, we recover and regain a normal, healthy vibration once again. We get over an incident or a remark and heal. But to do that successfully, we need *flexibility*—that is, the ability to flex, get unstuck, and regain health.

But what is *chronic* disease? That's when we get wedged in a state that we can't shake. It might be depression, anxiety, insomnia, chronic pain, asthma, cancer, or intransigent habits and addictions. In response, we do something that humans are very good at: we adapt to it. We forget that things were ever different. We accept the pronouncements of doctors that consign us to a disease category. (Indeed, such pronouncements are a big part of the problem.) We try to survive the rest of our lives on medication.

Another common method of adaptation is utilizing other types of "medication" to survive: alcohol, recreational drugs, and diversions like shopping, entertainment, and overeating. These things help to take our minds off our woes. Sometimes they can even be helpful. Binging on our favorite TV show can, at times, shift us out of our sadness or negativity and we can eventually lose our dependency on watching it. But more often, palliative drugs and diversions don't create a curative shift because we haven't really faced the root of our problem. Instead, we've just patched it over or avoided it.

So how can we heal? We need to regain flexibility again and get *unstuck*. Even medical professionals who hold conventional views about the body acknowledge the importance of flexibility. Consider your heart. You might think that a very regular heartbeat (or blood pressure) is a good thing. Not so! It's a sign of disease. A normal heartbeat is always slightly irregular. This variability and flexibility enables your heart to speed up and slow down as needed. The same goes for your blood pressure.

Flexibility is also required for emotional health. You might believe that someone who always remains calm, no matter what is happening, is healthier than a person with a more variable emotional state. Wrong! If a person doesn't have some kind of emotional reaction to tragedy, loss, or a joyful event, it's a sign of suppression of some kind. And as we will discuss later on in this book, suppression—especially to the point that a person is no longer even aware of his or her emotions—is a recipe for some very serious health problems.

That is precisely why the modern medical approach of artificially easing or suppressing every symptom does not usually achieve a lasting cure and can even be a recipe for more serious problems down the line.

If you lose your spouse, you are supposed to mourn, not simply pop an antidepressant or force yourself to act like nothing has happened. If you have bacteria causing havoc in your body, you are supposed to get a fever, whose very purpose is to wipe it out. After all, our bodies evolved to heal! In contrast, artificially suppressing every bit of life's sadness, every fever, and every flu symptom, disables the body from doing its job—healing itself and regaining a healthy vibrational state.

Of course, there are limits. If someone becomes wedged in mourning for years, or if a feverish patient heats up to the point that their life is in danger, other measures must be taken. But in general, the best way out is through. Allow your body and mind and emotions to do what they were designed to do naturally.

At this point you might be thinking: "But what if I'm in a chronic state of suffering and I can't recover? I can't survive this pain or sadness or anxiety any longer. I need drugs!"

Never fear. You're not on your own. Like I said, there are many tools out there besides conventional drugs and unhealthy diversions, and most of them can be combined with conventional treatments. They include meditation, self-introspection and releasing techniques (for example, the Sedona Method), energy-based therapies that work on a vibrational level (like homeopathy), psychological techniques like behavior modification therapy, hypnotherapy, or psychotherapy, structural methods like posture therapies and chiropractic, and many more. So, there's a lot of help available. And most of these approaches don't involve suppression or running away from a problem. Many can even be performed on your own, at no cost.

The trick is to find the tools that work for you and that address your problem at the level (or levels) at which it originates. Recently, this has been called "root-cause medicine." But the fact is, this approach to healing has been an important precept of alternative healing modalities for hundreds and even thousands of years. Indeed, the quest to find the root cause of disease, whether it be in the physical or energy bodies, is a big part of what this book is about.

I believe that for most health problems, true healing is a real possibility. But even if complete health and happiness isn't possible, a lot of improvement can be achieved. You *can* become happier, healthier, more successful, and more at peace. But it does take sincere effort. It's worth it, don't you think?

CHAPTER 2

᛭

WHAT IS
"LIVING IN SYNCHRONY"?

O f course, vibration isn't just something going on within us or intruding upon us from the outside. It's actually what we *interact* with every second of every day. Each of us is like a fish swimming in an ocean of vibration; we sense every wave coming our way, and we contribute our own waves into the mix. *Swimming with ease within this ocean is actually what "living in synchrony" is all about.* Moreover, because the ocean of vibration isn't just external to us but *one* with us—indeed, part of us—it deeply affects our bodies, emotions, minds, and spirit.

Most of us know what it feels like to be "in sync" with someone, some situation, or with the flow of life itself. Sometimes it is called "being in the zone." We sleep soundly, eat right, and feel energized. Amazing opportunities seem to fall into our laps. We easily partner up with just the right people. No problems as we sail through security at the airport, the cop lets us off with a warning, and our long-planned vacation is full of amazing adventures. On a deeper level, we feel in communion with a kind of energetic flow. We trust that everything will turn out right—and it does.

Most of the time, though, we operate as if the world were a big machine that we have little control over. We constantly try to fix things

17

that get broken or plan things in advance so that we don't get caught in the world's seemingly mechanical crunching gears. Rather than simply relaxing and *trusting*, we plan our vacations down to the minute or constantly check our smart phones to inspect every detail or change that comes our way. The same goes for our body—another elaborate "machine." We tune it up, pop another pill, and do everything the doctor says. We try to *force* ourselves to be well.

Deep down inside, though, we suspect that all of these pills and props and plans only go skin deep. Things may work out pretty well most of the time, but they can still get out of whack—even badly so. That's when we consider seeking the kind of help that operates at a deeper level. We may see a therapist, pray, meditate, or visit alternative healers who work at an energetic level of our being. We may find solace and support by engaging with others in a spiritual community or seek counsel with friends, family, or clergy.

If things get even more difficult, though, we may venture a bit more "out there" in our quest. We seek out a psychic or shaman. We look for omens and signs, utilize divination techniques like tarot cards or the I Ching, and try to pay more attention to subtle inspirations, intuitions, and dreams. When we do, we are operating under the assumption that there *is* a deeper order of reality that is truly the driver of our outer experience. Although we may forget about such things when our world gets more or less back on track, a new possibility may now exist for us, at least to some degree—that there *is* an expanded realm, beyond the veil of our supposedly machine-like lives. And we may begin to wonder in our quiet moments whether there might be something infinite and unknowable at work—the mind of God, if you will. There are signs all around us that indicate that this is true, if we just pay attention.

First, there are those uncanny synchronicities that pop into our lives, especially when something important happens. You might think of them as meaningful and often fortuitous "coincidences." However, as I will explain in the next chapter, the phenomenon of synchronicity is likely a fundamental property of vibrational reality; that is, that things with similar vibrational meaning tend to occur at the same time and place.

Here's one that occurred when I was taking my PhD oral qualifying exam, a part of my doctoral studies in computer science. Just at the moment when I realized that I didn't know the answer to a question a professor had asked me, the building's power went out! Not only was I "in the dark," but the building was too! When the exam was finally resumed, the difficult question was forgotten and omitted. Whew!

Or perhaps you've experienced an "aha!" moment when an insight suddenly occurs to you in the shower—an insight that leads you to make a big and ultimately positive change in your life. Or maybe you grudgingly decide to try some form of alternative medicine that "makes no sense" to you, but then you experience the cure of a lifelong chronic condition that all past efforts at treatment had failed to touch. Maybe you decide to visit a psychic medium and make contact with a deceased love one—and he or she provides you with information they could not possibly have known.

Are all such occurrences simply nonsense or coincidence? That's what we usually try to tell ourselves. We may be amazed for a day or two, but eventually we put it out of our minds. Life goes on as before. But when these occurrences are truly life changing or become more frequent, they become harder and harder to ignore. We begin to accept that there *must* be some deeper order, a more comprehensive reality. Several of my life's experiences have led me to that conclusion.

So again, what is *living in synchrony?* It's about getting in touch with this greater reality and learning to understand and even make use of its magic. I don't claim to have all the answers and I still get out of sync at times. But I truly believe that this deeper reality exists, not only because of my own experiences, but also because it aligns with so many systems of thought and wisdom that I have studied. This book will point you toward some of these resources so that you can begin to explore them on your own. If you do, you may discover that you slowly become more effective at actively participating with this magic.

Of course, very few humans (if any!) live in synchrony all the time. Perhaps even Jesus and Buddha got only part way there. But each of us can make progress if we make a little effort. The experiences of meditators and practitioners of healing strategies from around the world confirm that this is true. When we do, the rewards can be great: not only a healthier and less stressful life, but also greater happiness, trust, equanimity, and influence upon the evolution of our lives.

That's what living in synchrony is all about. *It's about lining up with what's going on within and without.* Internally, we line up with who we really are—our greater Self that encompasses not only our physical body, but also our thoughts, emotions, and energy bodies. Externally, we align with the greater outer reality of which we are a part—a reality in which we can function as true co-creators, and in which phenomena like synchronicities are fundamental and help to guide and enable our creations.

In essence, when you live in synchrony, you line up with what *is* rather than fighting, denying, or resisting it. And even when things aren't going exactly as you'd like, you more easily trust that everything is happening as it should and must. The reasons may not yet be obvious to you, but you have confidence that they will ultimately become clear.

Finally, consider this. Perhaps our global society's growing interconnection via the internet actually reflects a more profound interconnection that's also happening at unseen levels of reality. As the adage goes, "as above, so below"—or perhaps in this case, "as below, so above." Thus, instead of just connecting online, what if humanity is beginning to connect on all levels of our being, perhaps even connecting on all levels with the Earth's being? What if all of humanity could learn to live in synchrony? What if we could develop powerful shared psychic perceptions, dreams, and collective unitive states of consciousness?

I believe there are forces in the world today that would like to disrupt this deeper, energetic, and spiritual interconnectivity because they know the power it could yield would be truly awesome and ultimately uncontrollable. That is why protecting your *natural* humanity and your connection to this power is critical. And that is why learning to live in synchrony, within and without, may be more important now than ever.

CHAPTER 3

꒜

OPEN AND EXPAND
YOUR VIEW

Perhaps you've heard of the famous allegory or teaching story called "Plato's Cave." It's named after its author, the great Greek philosopher Plato, and it goes something like this. Imagine there are people living their entire lives inside a cave. Unfortunately, they are also shackled to chairs so that they face away from the light outside. Because of this, the only thing they can see is a play of shadows upon the cave wall. To them, this shadow play is their only known reality—flat images that merely hint at the true glory of nature lying just outside their reach. How can they become liberated so that they can see what's actually going on?

Plato utilized this allegory to suggest that humans are inherently limited by their own ignorance. But what if the cave allegory is actually closer to literal truth? Just like fish swimming in a fishbowl or Plato's people sitting in a cave, what if our perceptions are drastically limited by what we can sense? And what if a greater, deeper reality lies just beyond these limits?

We already know that many animals possess sense abilities that we humans do not. As a result, they live in a completely different "reality" than we do. For example, a dog's world is all about the vast panorama of smell—a world rich in odors that we cannot begin to imagine. It's really not that hard to consider that there *could* be realities we have not yet been able to detect, even with our best scientific instruments.

For instance, what if we are more than just our physical bodies, and, instead, are interpenetrated and surrounded by energy bodies that we cannot see with our physical senses? If so, what could these unseen parts of us enable us to sense and do? Do our minds actually reach beyond our limited boney skulls? These possibilities currently lie outside the sphere of conventionally accepted science, but they are definitely within the scope of the world's mystical traditions as well as frontier sciences that investigate things like psychic phenomena.[1]

We can also utilize Plato's lesson to understand common aspects of everyday experience. For example, when we were young, our families and hometown were all we knew. That was "the world" to us. But as we grew up, we understood that our limited child-view was only a small piece of a much larger picture. The same thing happens when we meet people who have different life experiences than our own, or when we watch movies about different times, places, and types of people. Slowly, we realize that, in many ways, we live in our own separate reality and perceive the world through our own unique lens—a lens that might be blocking out a great deal of information. We are literally held within a "cave" inundated by media, propaganda, advertising, our life experiences, our senses, the limits of accepted and acceptable knowledge, the pronouncements of authorities, and the philosophy of life deemed true by our society, religion, and family. And because we are so used to this "reality," adopting a new point of view can feel strange—even uncomfortable.

Today, this discomfort has become accentuated because "truth" has become harder and harder to discern. For instance, as mentioned in the introduction, many of us are starting to realize that once-trusted sources of information may be suspect because they are manipulated through censorship and other mechanisms that curate what we see or hear.

Interestingly, however, this situation may also be providing us with a unique opportunity for healing. Because in order for us to break free of many, if not most, physical and emotional ailments and transform our lives, we must examine our lenses and question our perception of what is really going on. In other words, the current state of the world is causing each of us to examine what is actually true.

Now, I'm not saying that we should repudiate all media and conventional science. I'm just saying we need to *expand* our view of reality and allow for the fact that there might be more going on beneath the surface than we realize. If we do, we may discover that there's a whole world outside our respective caves. In particular, we may understand more deeply the nature of who we are as complete human beings and why the various healing tools I describe in this book could be helpful to us.

WILL YOU CONSIDER AGE OLD WISDOM OR STICK TO MODERN CONVENIENCE?

Naturally, the proof of what I will describe in this book is ultimately "in the pudding"—that is, whether the ideas and healing methods based on an expanded world-view actually work in practice. Many of them are very old and have been helping people for thousands of years—much longer than modern medical science. Indeed, while today's "conventional" medicine seems to be always shifting and changing and often repudiates its own certainties and treatments just a few years after they are introduced, many of the techniques and modalities described in this book have remained much the same for hundreds and even thousands of years.

Some of what I will describe in Part II has even made its way, at least to some extent, into Western scientific philosophy. For example, the fields of psychiatry and, later, psychology, began with the realization that there is more going on within us than mere physical signs and symptoms. Fundamental to these fields was Sigmund Freud's "discovery" of the subconscious mind—a part of us that we are usually not aware of, but that affects the way we think, feel, and behave in very profound ways. For instance, our subconscious mind remembers all of the emotional pain of our childhood, even if it is blocked from our day-to-day adult awareness. By uncovering and working with this hidden part of us, remarkable cures can be achieved.

Freud's student Carl Jung expanded upon Freud's initial work and took it to some quite esoteric places. In particular, he discovered an even deeper truth about our collective reality: that there is a realm of *meaning* within the universe that affects not only our minds and emotions, but physical occurrences in our environment too. He called this phenomenon *synchronicity*—the co-occurrence of events in space and time that are connected by meaning. Synchronicities are what we sometimes call "meaningful coincidences."

As an illustration of the phenomenon, Jung pointed out that it is no mere accident that a man's watch stops ticking the moment he dies, or that an insect appears in a room just as a patient is describing a dream about that same type of insect. Jung hypothesized that these synchronicities occur because, at a deeper level, meaning *creates* reality. If this is true, we too must be creators, and not simply because of our physical actions. Our dreams, thoughts, and emotions may actually be creating events in our lives. As a result, we are not simply biological robots buffeted about in a random world of chance (the modern scientific view), but instead, are co-creators in an infinitely complex expanded reality that is affected by energies within fields of meaning.

Unfortunately, in the late 20th century, psychology and especially psychiatry veered away from Jung's profound insights. His ideas became an embarrassment to a field that wanted desperately to be accepted as modern and "scientific." As a result, psychology and psychiatry began to focus on elaborations of the "man-as-biological-robot" theme. Lab rats were run around mazes in controlled experiments, based on the assumption that humans are just like lab rats too. The emerging field of computer science (my own field of study) further exacerbated this tendency to understand humans as biological computers.

Sadly, the mysteries of the subconscious mind are largely ignored by today's psychiatrists and even by some psychologists. They have been influenced by the immense power of the pharmaceutical industry, which encourages doctors to hand out pills instead of utilizing more traditional talk-therapy. Now, even children are hooked on meds for their emotional and behavioral problems. It's the new normal. What are the physical, emotional, and behavioral consequences of this strategy down the line?

THE IMPERATIVE OF FRONTIER SCIENCE

Despite all of this, there does seem to be a growing societal interest in a more nuanced and deeper view of reality. Many of us are feeling disillusioned with the limited vistas that conventional science, medicine, and mainstream society offer us. We may intuitively sense that there *is* more going on, and we are delving into ancient forms of wisdom, the practice of meditation, and even the use of hallucinogens to access new states of awareness. That's why there are a growing number of workshops being offered that teach things like how to have out-of-body experiences, engage in lucid dreaming, communicate with plants, and more.

Are all of these so-called "New Age" explorations an escape into fantasy and wishful thinking? In some cases and for some people, yes. But they also indicate that people are opening up to the possibility that commonly held views about what reality is should be expanded. As I discuss in much more detail in my book *Active Consciousness,* there is an emerging group of frontier scientists who utilize the methods of modern science to *prove* the existence of an expanded reality. I have had the opportunity to meet some of them, and my husband Steve, also a computer scientist, helped a few of them implement their research experiments.

Consider, for example, the studies conducted by Dean Radin, PhD, chief scientist of the Institute of Noetic Sciences (IONS) in Petaluma, California. Over the years, Radin's controlled experiments have demonstrated some remarkable things: that humans can anticipate what will happen before it occurs; that connected couples' body readings synchronize even when they are shielded from one another in sealed rooms; that mass events where people are experiencing similar emotions can affect the behavior of machines. In one experiment, fifty machines scattered all over the world began to veer away from their normal behavior just *before* the World Trade Center towers were hit on 9/11. Radin has gone on to do many more studies of this kind, as have other scientists at IONS.[2]

Or consider the work of Russell Targ on remote viewing. Targ's work, funded by the US Department of Defense in the 1970s and 1980s, demonstrated that each of us may have the ability to "see" things at a distance. Particularly skilled individuals were even able to remotely view secret military facilities in the USSR while they were sitting in Targ's laboratory in California—information that was verified years later. Targ also demonstrated that we may be able to sense things that occurred in the past or will occur in the future. That is, time and distance don't seem to make a difference when we use an expanded version of our sensing abilities.[3]

Another pioneer in frontier science is biologist Rupert Sheldrake, who has focused on understanding how people, animals, and even minerals can communicate with one another despite a lack of any scientifically accepted means of interaction. For example, difficult-to-synthesize crystals become easier to crystallize over time at distant locations—even if information about the process is not communicated between laboratories. Sheldrake's experiments also demonstrated that pets can sense information about their owners at large distances.[4]

How is all of this possible? Sheldrake hypothesizes that an unseen field, which he calls the *morphic field,* interpenetrates our reality and enables such communications to occur—especially if the communicating people, animals, or even plants and minerals have already come into contact with one another or are part of the same species or some other kind of grouping. That's why the couples in Radin's experiments were able to synchronize with one another even when they were sealed into separate compartments. And that's how animals find their owners who have moved thousands of miles away.

Sheldrake also hypothesizes that it is the morphic field that holds our thoughts and memories, not our physical brains. Just as a radio or TV broadcast is held in the "airwaves" and is received by a radio or TV set, our brains may simply be receivers that pick up our thoughts and memories stored in the morphic field. You might think of this information as being available on various channels of vibration, much like TV channels. Our own personal channel, storing all of our own memories, is the one we receive the best. Next easiest to "tune into" might be the channel we share with family and friends. A bit harder (but not impossible) to pick up might be the channel we share with our town, our nation, and our species. Perhaps that is what Jung meant by the "collective unconscious." Physicists already agree that subatomic particles can become *entangled* so that they are able to communicate and coordinate their behaviors at a distance. If Sheldrake is correct, we humans and everything else around us may be entangled too.

A REVOLUTION IS COMING

Most scientists tend to repudiate all of these frontier studies as hogwash, and there is good reason for them to do so. Accepting this research would force them to question much of their life's work. On top of this, society would, in many ways, be upended by the acceptance of such ideas.

The truth is, huge revolutions in world-view have always been met by formidable opposition. Hundreds of years ago, frontier scientists like Radin, Targ, and Sheldrake were persecuted and sometimes even executed for saying that the Earth wasn't flat or that it orbited around the sun. As the famous story goes, Galileo's peers refused to look through his telescope to see whether there were moons revolving around Jupiter. For them, this possibility was threatening and simply "impossible." Their world-views were strictly limited and guarded; they *wanted* to remain in the cave.

But with time, the truth has a tendency to leak out and eventually become accepted. It may take a lot of time, though—even centuries. We may no longer kill people who promulgate new views of reality, but the power of money and media are still very effective at censoring and marginalizing them. Their TedX lectures are removed online (this happened to both Targ and Sheldrake). Similarly, medical information that threatens the pharmaceutical industry (like studies that prove the efficacy of homeopathic remedies, or reveal the disturbing contents of the US government's growing database of vaccine injuries) is ignored or dismissed by the media and "disappeared" from online search engines. Why? Because big money has big power. In fact, practitioners of unconventional healing methods are routinely denied research grants and sometimes lose their right to practice.

Ultimately, we need patience. A change to our collective view of reality will happen gradually, at least at first. A small group of people who see things in a new way may share their views and gain some followers. There may be attempts to repress or censor them, followed by an eventual rebirth of interest in their ideas. Gradually, the new view will become acceptable. Pieces then become co-opted and integrated into the mainstream.

As an illustration, there are many more people interested in meditation now than there used to be, largely because scientific studies have proven that it can improve brain and emotional health. Many of these modern-day meditators don't believe in the spiritual ideas about different realities and past lives that are part and parcel of the traditions that pioneered such practices. Likewise, researchers who measure the brain waves of meditating Buddhist priests usually aren't interested in the insights the priests have while meditating. Nevertheless, it's progress.

Eventually, however, the group that accepts a new world-view grows large enough so that a tipping-point is reached. That's the point at which this view becomes mainstream and former views are repudiated. Some believe we may be nearing such a tipping-point. In fact, philosopher Ken Wilber has pointed out that one sign of an impending shift is that there are more and more attacks on the new world-view.[5] We are certainly experiencing that today, especially leading up to, during, and after the COVID years.

For instance, consider the recent treatment of homeopathic medicine by the media and governmental bodies. This form of alternative treatment was once a mainstream form of medicine in the United States, largely due to its success in treating epidemics. Unfortunately, it was squashed by conventional allopathic medicine in the early and mid 1900s due to the rising power of the pharmaceutical industry. During the 1970s, however, homeopathy began to make a comeback, especially because of its success in treating chronic disease. Today, because homeopathic remedies have become increasingly popular, the FDA is trying to outlaw them. Ironically, the legislation that established the FDA in the first place was written by Senator Royal Copeland, who was also a homeopathic doctor! Copeland enshrined into the FDA legislation various guarantees that protected homeopathic medicine as a distinct and protected category. Now, the FDA is busy dismantling these guarantees.

Or consider the fact that in mid 2019, just before the COVID years began, online search engines like Google began demoting sites that promote alternative views on health and diet—even the use of vitamins to mitigate disease. The highest-ranking alternative health site on the internet, Mercola.com, was essentially removed from view overnight.

Several years before that, though, information about almost every form of alternative medicine on Wikipedia was completely corrupted by so-called quackbusters. Every effort to correct this information has been stymied.

Will a fundamental shift in world view about these kinds of subjects lose its momentum and be halted? Will the corporate-funded powers have their way? It's too soon to say. One goal of this book is to keep the momentum building, at least in the area of health. The payoff for those who adopt a new world-view is huge—escaping enslavement to the medical machine and finding new ways to heal. In a world where health care costs are astronomical and many conventional approaches no longer work or are more harmful than helpful, we may not have a choice.

What You Will Find in This Book

In Part II, I will begin my presentation of an expanded view of who and what we are. In essence, it is a scientific hypothesis that unifies much of what I've learned from many teachings and healing approaches. It might be viewed as a cosmology that answers questions about the nature of life and death. Unlike many writers in this genre, however, I don't focus on any one particular approach or philosophy. Instead, I try to combine many ideas together. The result is something that fits most such teachings while removing some of their low-level details. Personally, I find this approach to be not only more compelling and clarifying, but also easier to accept and believe. But it also means that I am always refining my ideas as I learn more. As I describe these ideas in the chapters that follow, I'll also provide fictional scenarios that help illustrate them.

After Part II comes Part III—a description of tools and methodologies that can help you to heal. They are organized according to the model developed in Part II—in particular, the many layers that comprise our being. Yes, we have a physical body, and it includes structures and mechanisms still being uncovered by medical science. There is also the whole world of bacteria, fungi, and other microbiota dwelling within and around us. This microscopic realm is a new and growing field of science, and it deeply affects and interacts with our physical and emotional health.

But then it goes deeper. Interpenetrating the physical body and its microbiota are energy fields that regulate and control how all of these physical, chemical, and microscopic entities are working. This is the realm of energy-based medicines like homeopathy, acupuncture, and hands-on healing. Beyond that are even more esoteric aspects of our being. I believe these deeper levels exist before and after our physical life here on Earth. How do they affect us? Can we communicate with, learn from, and heal them too? Yes.

Once we accept this layered view of who and what we are, it becomes fairly obvious that the tools we need to best heal and transform ourselves will be determined by *where* the crux of any particular problem lies. For example, if someone's leg is broken in an accident, they will definitely need to visit a medical doctor and have it put into a cast. After that, other modalities like homeopathy, acupuncture, or the use of herbs may help the bone to heal faster. By exploring even more deeply, however, the patient might be able to comprehend *why*, at a deeper level, they may have broken their leg in the first place. Is it possible that the accident was triggered by a deeper soul-level goal, say, of promoting emotional growth? Often, only a retrospective view on life can yield such answers.

In any case, none of the tools and methodologies described in Part III will make sense to you if you cannot accept their viability. Nor will you be willing to utilize them. That's why it's important to expand your view—so that you can get out of your cave, open your eyes to what may really be going on, and then utilize a wider set of options for growth and healing.

IT GOES BEYOND PERSONAL HEALING

Truthfully, these concepts can go way beyond personal healing. They apply to our local, national, and global society too. They apply to all of the living things on Earth and to the Earth itself. They may even apply to the solar system, galaxy, and universe! All of the realms described in Part II exist on an interconnected energetic level, even if we cannot see or sense them. And all are affected by fields of meaning, synchronicities, and more.

Many of us are reeling from the changes that the COVID years brought upon us. The future feels increasingly uncertain. Will society become ever more compartmentalized, surveilled, and controlled by powerful entities that limit what we can and cannot do, where we can and cannot go? Will we be funneled into a future in which humans are cajoled or forced to merge with machines or become genetically modified, turning us into so-called "transhumans"? Many people, especially my old colleagues in Silicon Valley, eagerly look forward to this future and believe it is our human destiny.

As you might have guessed by now, I vehemently disagree. The transhumanistic urge is predicated on the notion that we *are* simply biological machines. Those who embrace this view believe that by augmenting themselves through gene-editing and AI-based technology, they can become super-biological machines, possibly even immortal. But the transhumanists of Silicon Valley are barking up the wrong tree. Their premise is fundamentally misguided. We *aren't* just biological machines. *We are already superhumans, intrinsically connected to an energetic universe that we just haven't fully tapped into yet.*

Spreading this truth is one of the main reasons I was motivated to complete this book. I believe that if we tamper with our very real and natural human selves, we may wind up cutting ourselves off from untapped power. Just as Delilah disempowered Goliath by cutting his hair, editing our genes or merging ourselves with AI may cut us off from our deeper spiritual potential and connection.

The COVID years gave us an initial bitter taste what might be coming our way. The more we are cut off from each other, the more we live our lives in virtual realities, and the more we are monitored and controlled, the less fully human we become. I believe that the result will be disastrous. Not only will our physical health be harmed or crippled (necessitating, of course, even more drugs and external props in order to survive), but our planetary civilization may ultimately wither and die. *It's time to wake up and embrace our powerful, natural, self-healing, complete Selves!* I hope this book helps you to understand this message more deeply and how urgent the situation may truly be.

PART II

WHAT'S REALLY GOING ON?

"We are complete in ourselves; and the reason why we fail to realize this
is that we do not understand how far the 'self' of ourselves extends...
Walt Whitman was quite right when he said that we are not all included
between our hat and our boots."
– **Thomas Troward**

CHAPTER 4

﹥

THE BOX

Each of us spends a great deal of our life living in a box. I'm not talking about houses or apartments. I'm talking about our internal boxes—*our minds*. Most of the time, these "mind-boxes" seem to have impenetrable steel walls. We can look within, but the mysteries lying inside another person's mind-box remain ultimately unknowable. When we take the time to examine the contents of our own box, we discover words, pictures, and even the sounds of our thoughts, reverberating and echoing, bouncing and triggering one another, in a never-ending stream of chatter and imagery.

The most commonly accepted scientific view of the mind is that it is all a matter of brain waves and neurons firing, which trigger the rush of chemicals we sense as emotions, aches, pains, and pleasurable sensations in our bodies. We are told that we humans (and all other living things) are simply biological machines, albeit pretty amazing ones, and that our sense of "self"—who we are, what we believe and experience, from the color and smell of a rose to the most exotic hallucination or meditative insight—is just a byproduct of neurons firing in our brains. Any other notion that we might have about ourselves is tossed off as wishful thinking or self-aggrandizing delusion.

Upon further examination, you will notice that your mind-box also has boxes within it. When you read a book or watch a movie or TV show, you experience the feeling of being embedded in yet *another* world. These more interior worlds can often take precedence over your perceptions of the physical world around you. Just walk down any busy street and you will find people staring down at yet another little box in their hands. Sometimes it seems like people barely know what's going on in their physical environment anymore. I've been nearly mowed down on a sidewalk more than once by a smartphone user whose primary residence has become the virtual world of the internet.

Sadly, the proliferation of smart phones in our world has quickly had a profound impact on our connection to outer reality. The consequences of living this way are only beginning to be felt. What will it mean if humanity completely cuts itself off from its physical environment—even parents from their own children? Studies now show that parents who are distracted by their smartphones do not interact normally with their infants and toddlers, and as a result, are causing damage to their children's cognitive development.[1] What will be the impact in ensuing generations?

The COVID years produced an intensification of this phenomenon and served as a rehearsal for a potentially ominous future. Lockdowns and vaccine mandates isolated us from friends and family, turning us into solitary creatures forced to interact via computer screens. Our bodies literally became boxes wrapped in protective coverings that didn't allow us to breathe freely. One of my "wake up" moments during COVID occurred when a participant in a spiritual group I had been part of (naturally, now online) announced that she intended to wear a mask for the rest of her life. In my experience, those living in highly technocentric environments like Silicon Valley are highly susceptible to a fear and self-protection ethos. During COVID, many became agoraphobic addicts to their boxes, and many are still living that way, years later.

Now, I'm not saying that the virtual world of the internet is all bad. As I said before, I used to be a researcher in computer science—in the field of artificial intelligence no less. So I can understand the allure and utility of the virtual world. Many aspects of those virtual boxes within our mind-boxes are truly marvelous. Through them, we can be connected, via the wonders of electronics and telecommunication, to nearly anyone on the planet, at any time of day. We can gain access to seemingly infinite information and entertainment merely by asking for it. It's completely addictive—and that's the problem. No wonder an increasing number of people are spending most of their lives inside this box-in-a-box. But at what price? Are the wonders afforded to us by the virtual world—especially if they remain unchecked—really worth it? Are we, as a society, truly happy? Are *you* truly happy?

STOP THE CHATTER AND LOOK WITHIN

While humanity was busy developing technology—from the wheel to the smart phone—every civilization on Earth was also on a quest to find the keys to true happiness, contentment, and fulfillment. Yes, the development of technology was part of that. But within each civilization, the wise ones tended to focus on meaning rather than money, on enlightenment rather than on entertainment or comfort. Those who were successful discovered that the best strategy was to become aware of what lies beyond the echoing chamber of their mind-box.

All of us know that we become more relaxed when we turn off our electronics, drop the daily newspaper, and simply lie on a beach or some other place in nature. We become happier as we freely breathe fresh air and listen to the waves as they hit the shore, the leaves rustling in the breeze, or the uniquely soothing sound of birdsong. One of the reasons for this is that the natural environment enables our physical senses to take precedence over our mind-boxes. Nature reengages us with the air, soil, water, plants, animals, and other energies in which we evolved as human beings. Thrill seekers who pursue extreme sports or gain a sense of aliveness by putting themselves in dangerous situations also experience the relief of being in the moment, all senses alive and attuned.

But you don't need to go bungee jumping or climb a mountain to become happier. A much less strenuous and more cost-effective way to tame your addiction to your busy mind-box is *meditation*. By using a variety of techniques—focusing on one's breath, settling into body sensation, repeating a mantra, or gazing at an object—practitioners of meditation can relieve the stress and sufferings of daily life by simply quieting the busy echo chambers of their minds. Dialing down this internal hubbub takes them into the present moment—the *Now*. And in the Now, there *is* no worry, no fear, no regret, no stories, no cravings, and no suffering.

In the Now, we also become more aware of our surroundings and the beauty of life all around us—the sounds of nature, the wind on our cheeks, the yearning of a growing blade of grass or flower, and yes, the wonders of technology too. Instead of needing to run to a forest, we feel content and grateful right where we are. Scientific studies have even demonstrated that meditating, for just ten-minutes a day, can rebuild brain tissue.[2] As a result, even conventional scientists are beginning to acknowledge that quieting the chatter inside our minds is healthy for our brains, just as sleep is important for our physical bodies.

But is that all there is to it? De-stressing, resting, and building new brain tissue? As you might guess, these benefits are just the tip of an iceberg. Although modern science generally refuses to look beyond these benefits, thousands of years of wisdom and teachings developed by meditators from all over the world reveal that much more can be gained.

That is when things get interesting, and certainly problematic for anyone of a strictly materialistic bent. In the past, the kind of knowledge that could be gained by journeying within was kept secret by shamans and mystics. Today, however, more and more people are realizing that a quieted mind, resting in the Now, is a gateway to an expanded realm of human awareness, experience, and ability. Being in the Now is just the first step toward dissolving the steel walls of our mind-boxes and entering a new world of possibilities—*a world in which receiving information and insights, perceiving different parallel realities, and developing an ability to more deeply understand and exert a greater influence upon our own reality, become commonplace.*

Think of it this way. Normally, we aren't even paying attention to what's going on in the echo chamber of our minds. It's like being on a noisy street or in a crowded restaurant; it's hard to make out the individual sounds or notice the small things, so we don't even try. But when we meditate and our minds become quieter, we slow things down and begin to notice what's going on. Occasional thoughts drift by and become more discernable. Sensations are more deeply felt and sounds are more acutely heard. If you meditate with your eyes open—yes, you can do that and I often prefer it—you will find that the world around you becomes much more vivid. And as things become even quieter, more things start to happen.

First, you actually begin to *notice* your box. You become its observer, and you become aware that you are doing so. This is the point at which you have achieved what is sometimes called the "observer state." This step alone can be transformational, because it breaks down your identification with your thoughts and feelings. If you can observe what's going on inside your box, you realize that *you* aren't its contents. Chronic worries about the future or feelings of anger or sadness about the past become seen for what they are—thoughts and stories inside your box. As a result, you can detach from them a bit more easily. You can also become more objective and learn to modify your stories and your responses to them.

In contrast, if you have never realized that you aren't merely the sum total of your thoughts and feelings, you will never even entertain this possibility. You won't try to direct your thoughts and feelings because you believe they *are* you. Your thoughts and emotions just seem to overtake you and you feel powerless to do anything about them.

Here's an example of the utility of achieving the observer state. Suppose you are a chronic worrier (as I myself tend to be). If you try to catch yourself and notice when a worry surfaces in your mind—for instance, about your health—say to yourself (or even better, say out loud): "Oh, there I go, worrying about my health again!" or "STOP!". This step alone can help to dissipate a worry. And even if it doesn't, you can sit down for a few minutes, quiet your mind, and ease your worry through a variety of meditation techniques.

However, I do want to emphasize that gaining greater awareness of and control over your mind-box is not about suppressing your thoughts and feelings or punishing yourself for having them. In fact, it's quite the opposite. One teacher in this area is Tara Brach.[3] Her teaching of "RAIN" encapsulates this point. "RAIN" stands for **R**ecognize what is happening; **A**llow the experience to be there; **I**nvestigate with interest and care; and **N**urture with self-compassion. In other words, when you can see your mind-box for what it is, you can more easily develop self-acceptance and a deepened compassion for yourself. You become more compassionate towards others too. After all, they are also trapped in their mind-boxes. Thus, becoming the observer and eventual master of your mind-box is more about love and transcendence than force and control.

BEYOND THE BOX

Alleviating your suffering by becoming aware and observant of your thoughts and feelings is a huge step. It can result in a happier and more peaceful life. But if you stick with it, things can get even more interesting.

Once you've learned to quiet your box and take better hold of its contents, *the box itself begins to change*. Its walls begin to soften in texture, become more porous or transparent, and eventually begin to disappear. Not only do you begin to realize that you aren't the content of your box, but that a whole new world lies *outside* your box—a world you now have access to. That's because there is a part of you that *always* resides outside your mind-box; you are already a much more expansive being than you realize! You've simply been blocking your access to these parts of yourself. It's like seeing what's outside Plato's cave. It's discovering who and what you really are.

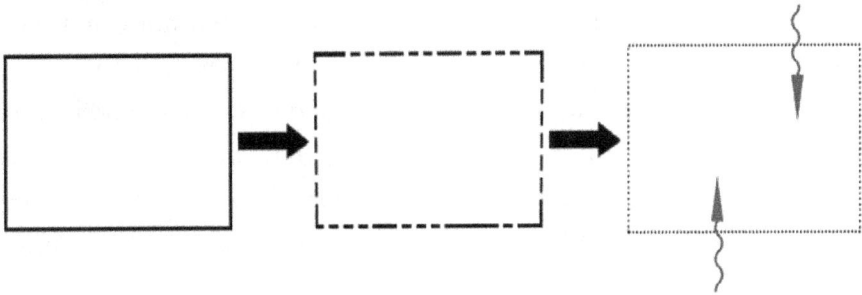

There are basically two kinds of things that happen to people who venture along this path. One is an expansion in perception and sensation. For example, you might begin to see aspects of the human energy field or aura. Or you might start experiencing more gut feelings about things—premonitions of events, or increased sensitivity and perception of other people's thoughts and emotions. Such abilities are often associated with people we call "psychic." There have even been children who have been trained (through the use of blindfolds and reinforcement techniques) to literally *see* their environment—even read a book—while blindfolded![4] They have achieved this ability by developing a visual sense that goes beyond their physical eyes.

Another thing that can happen at this stage is that conceptual information from outside your box is more easily received—perhaps sudden insights, artistic or scientific inspirations, or revelatory dreams. At first, these experiences may appear as brief snips or glimpses. You might be sitting in meditation, taking a shower, or staring at some clouds, and suddenly a new insight or idea pops into your head. It won't seem like anything you reasoned out. Instead, it will feel as if a small gap appeared in the steel walls of your mind and something poured in from the outside. Such moments of *in*-spiration or *in*-sight are usually accompanied by a sensation of increased energy, joy, and happiness.

Great scientists like Einstein, inventors like Tesla, and many artists, musicians and writers all report that their inspirations and new ideas often "come" to them when they aren't thinking about anything in particular. In those moments, the boxes of their minds became less noisy and their walls became a bit more porous, allowing something new to pop in. The wonderful thing is that such moments and experiences aren't confined to creative geniuses. We all have them. In fact, they are a natural part of being human. *We only need to expect them, learn how to recognize them, and pay attention to them.* When we do, they will begin to appear more frequently and more easily.

Naturally, it can sometimes be hard to distinguish between true insight and wishful or even delusional thinking. But once you have had an authentic experience of this kind and the information you receive is verified in some way, you will begin to know the difference. Like I said, there is often a distinct sensation in your body when an inspiration occurs—a spontaneous feeling of knowing, joy, and peace; an enlivening, energizing feeling. And the more you engage with this ability, the more your box and its walls will dissolve. Those who are adept receivers become our great wisdom-keepers and mystics.

If all of this sounds rather crazy and spooky, rest assured that no matter how much progress you make, your brain-mind and mind-box will remain intact. After all, you need them to navigate the physical world! That's why we evolved to have a brain and mind-box in the first place. However, when you start experiencing these new forms of awareness, you will also gain access to a much *greater* world—a reality that makes the virtual world of the internet seem like a mere board game.

After you open your box a bit, alternative healing modalities will also start to make more sense to you. Indeed, experiencing a profound healing from a medical system based upon an expanded view of what a human being really is—especially if this healing is considered "impossible" from the standpoint of conventional medicine—can itself be the trigger that starts the opening process. I know this was true for me and for the rest of my family when we discovered homeopathy.

So ask yourself: *Do you have any evidence that what I'm suggesting is true?* Begin by examining your own personal experiences.

For instance, nearly all of us have had some kind of psychic premonition—when we suddenly know who is going to call on the phone, or get one of those gut feelings that turned out to be correct. And even if you don't think you are the least bit psychic, you will probably acknowledge that small, spontaneous insights and inspirations do occasionally appear—often while you are in a reverie or perhaps while you are dreaming. Sometimes they occur as we awaken in the morning, or when we rest in a twilight state of openness. These pieces of received wisdom usually get lost in the chaos of our mind-boxes, and we simply ignore or forget them. Indeed, it's often only when the insights are extremely vivid and *can't* be ignored that we begin to notice them at all. But if you start to pay attention and keep a lookout for them, you may discover that they happen almost every day.

The truth is, receiving information and insight from your more complete Self is a natural part of being human, just as seeing with your eyes and feeling with your fingers are natural functions of your physical body. Such abilities are an intrinsic aspect of your full being. Developing access to them takes dedication, practice, and experimentation, but nearly everyone can make headway. So let's get started by learning more about what this more complete Self is all about.

CHAPTER 5

✶

WHO ARE WE?
WHAT ARE WE?

Let's get down to basics. Who are we? What are we?

First and foremost, we are more than just our physical bodies. Yes, our brains are involved in creating our perceptions and thoughts, but most of us intuitively sense that something more is going on. What *is* this something? Is it an unseen part of us—our soul or spirit—that goes on after we die?

In this chapter, I'll begin to answer these questions. My ideas about this topic have evolved after several years of reading and exploration. They combine my own experiences and intuitions with information provided by several teachers, mystics, and ancient traditions. My sources include Rudolph Steiner, G.I. Gurdjieff, Barbara Brennan, the teachings of Huna, the material taught by the International Academy of Consciousness (IAC), the discoveries of psychologist Michael Newton about the afterlife, the beliefs embraced by mystical traditions of many world religions, and more. You can research these sources on your own by exploring the various notes and references provided at the end of this book.

Personally, I think the fact that so many people from so many cultures and times have come to basically the same conclusions lends

46

credence to them. Just like the proverb about the blind men who each describe what they think an "elephant" is, each teacher or tradition provides a fragment of the complete picture. Some of the details might differ, but the general gestalt of the unified picture can slowly be discerned. It has been one of my goals in life to tease out this picture and share it with everyone. But this also means that whenever I learn something new, I expand and tweak the picture some more, striving to make it clearer and truer over time.

Of course, one of the best tests of any model or philosophy is its practical utility. If we are more than just our physical bodies, then it makes sense that disease and cure is also not limited to the physical. Can effective systems of healing be rooted in techniques that don't rely on the manipulation of bodily tissues and chemicals? Can human beings achieve feats of healing that would be impossible if we were just physical in nature? More and more evidence (as well as thousands of years of human experience) suggests that the answer is: *Yes.*

One of the main reasons I decided to write this book is to help you understand that it is quite likely that most of the ailments we suffer from are not rooted in the physical body at all. Yes, we experience symptoms in our bodies that are real and troublesome. But rather than patching them up with pills and potions that can only operate on a physical level, actually *curing* disease requires us to address it at its origin. In order for that to happen, we need to understand what's really going on.

Most of time we live as if we were simply physical bodies buffeted about in a world of cause and effect, and beyond that, pure chance. The events we experience often seem beyond our control. We feel like we are just one more billiard ball knocked around on the table of life. That view is also current scientific doctrine, and modern culture inculcates it within us in a million different ways. But what if there really is a lot more going on beneath the apparent physical surface? What if the dance of life is infinitely more subtle and intricate than we can imagine? For instance, what if everything we experience is influenced by our thoughts?

What if undetectable forces are at play that can alter the trajectory of our experienced reality in unexpected ways? If so, why not learn to play a more conscious role in this ballet of vibrating energy?

THE ENERGY BODY ARCHITECTURE

The truth is, our physical body is only a small part of our larger complete Self. The figure below illustrates how many teachers describe it. An actual depiction of who and what we are as seen from an even higher—perhaps higher-dimensional—perspective is likely even more complex and different. I'll discuss that more in Chapter 11. But for now, the figure below is a great place to start.

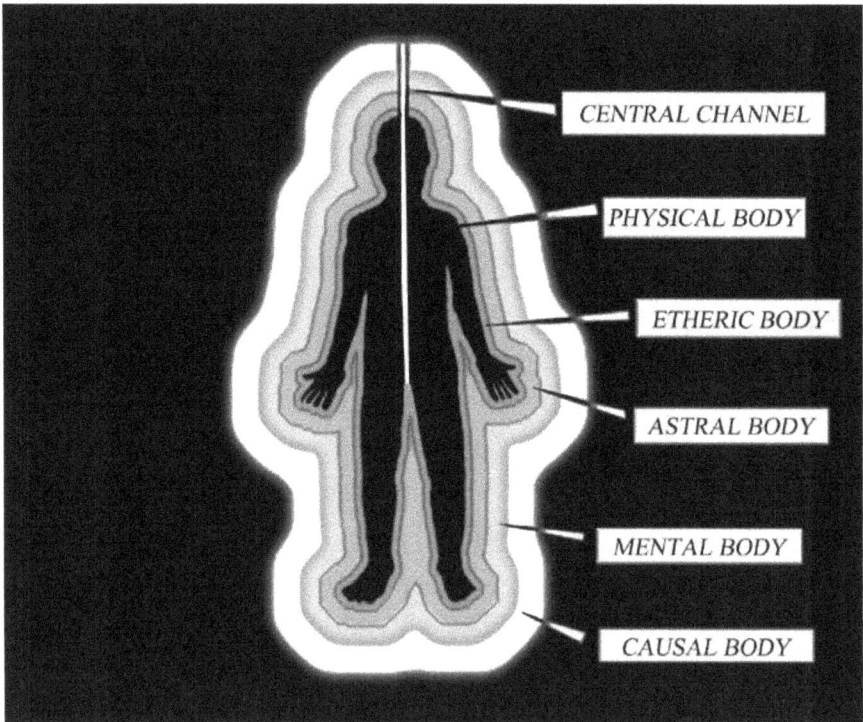

Each of us is composed of several layers or parts. The part that we experience most directly is the Physical Body, depicted as the black figure in the center. Beyond the physical—and interpenetrating it—are the various *energy bodies:* the Etheric, Astral, Mental, and Causal Bodies. (Note: the terms I've used in this book for the energy bodies are the ones commonly-used in English, but there are analogs in most languages and cultures.)

We may not see or feel our energy bodies (at least most of the time), but they are always with us. They affect our physical, emotional, mental, and spiritual experiences. Let's consider the Etheric Body first.

The Etheric Body

The first layer beyond the physical is often called the *Etheric Body*. The energy comprising this level has been called by many names—*chi, prana, vital force,* and more. People who can see the energy bodies (which is sometimes called the human "aura") describe the Etheric Body as having a bluish color, but other colors can be seen as well. Those who can see the etheric realm claim that all living things have Etheric Bodies—plants and animals, but perhaps minerals too.

Because the etheric level is the one closest to the physical, it is also the energy body that is the easiest to see and feel. In fact, I can sometimes see the Etheric Body if I am in certain kinds of lighting and in the right state of mind. Why not try to do so yourself? A typical beginner's exercise is to try to feel the chi between your hands. Hold your hands in front of you with palms facing each other, about six inches apart. Close your eyes. Now very slowly, move your palms toward each other. Do you notice a slight tingling sensation or a feeling of density or pressure? Play with this sensation by moving your hands slowly toward and away from each other. Can you notice the sensation of chi at further distances? You may even notice a taffy-like pulling sensation as the chi between your hands meets, blends, and then pulls apart.

Now try to *see* the etheric level. Go outside on a brightly lit day, sit, and settle yourself. Ideally, meditate for a while. Gaze at the trees. Can you see a bluish or grayish glow around them? Can you see cords of blue-gray energy reaching between the auras of two branches that are near one another?

Now, with a clear sky in the background, put your two hands in front of you, palms facing you and your fingertips reaching toward one another but not touching. Let your eyes defocus just a bit and try not to censor your experience. Be open. You may begin to see a bluish-gray aura around your fingers. Can you also see energy cords reaching between the fingers of your two hands? For me, these cords often appear yellow or rainbow-colored. Now, slowly move one of your hands upwards and see if these cords "stretch" as your fingertips move away from one another. If you can see this effect, it may convince you that what you are seeing is not an optical illusion, but rather, some form of energy that's always there; you just don't perceive it most of the time. Unless you are a particularly gifted aura reader, these visual perceptions will disappear as soon as you return to normal awareness.

So, what is the role of the etheric layer of our being? If animals and plants also have Etheric Bodies, it must be very fundamental to life.

In my view, our Etheric Body is a form of energy that radiates from our Physical Body—just like the magnetic field surrounding a magnet. However, the manipulation of the Etheric Body's energy can also cause profound changes in the Physical Body; it's a two-way street. In other words, the Etheric Body is not just a *byproduct* of the Physical Body; it is an intrinsic and independent aspect of who we are. There is even evidence that the Etheric Body continues to exist, at least for a while, after the Physical Body dies or pieces of it are removed. *Kirlian photography* was developed by Semyon Kirlian in the 1930s and is able to capture an image of the etheric layer. Amazingly, Kirlian's photographs of leaves revealed that after a leaf is cut, the Etheric Body of the cut-off portion is still visible, at least for a while.

The Etheric and Physical Bodies are constantly interacting and affecting one another in complex ways. Because of this, many alternative systems of healing focus on addressing the etheric level. Indeed, *they view the Etheric Body as the foundation and prime controller of the Physical Body*. If this is true, treating disease purely on a physical level cannot fully cure it. For example, even if a tumor or growth is cut out of the body, there may still be dysfunction on the etheric level that recreates the problem again. As we all know, physical disease often reoccurs in this way.

In general, healing systems that focus on the Etheric Body (like acupuncture, homeopathy, and hands-on healing) attempt to manipulate etheric energy in some way. By treating dysfunction at the etheric level, these therapies are able, as a downstream effect, to create fundamental and permanent change in the Physical Body. That's how homeopathy (my own area of expertise) is able to cure chronic diseases that conventional medicine can only palliate or alleviate. It is also interesting to note that the experience of healing at the etheric level usually doesn't feel the same as physically-based healing. Unlike physical treatments that essentially force the body to change, etheric healing is more subtle; it's as if a piece of information is being transmitted to the Etheric Body in order to nudge it out of its "stuckness." Once this happens, the Physical Body can use its own healing powers to correct itself. This will be discussed in much more detail in Chapter 15.

The innate power of the Etheric Body over the Physical Body also underlies many of the Asian disciplines that have the word "chi" or "ki" in their name—for example, martial arts like Tai Chi and Aikido, and healing exercises like Chi Gong. The etheric energy utilized, circulated, and enhanced by these practices is what enables a physically tiny martial artist to vanquish a physically stronger foe. It is also emanations from the Etheric Body of a healing guru that enable the physical cure of people who sit in their presence.

The Central Channel

If etherically-based medical philosophies are correct, not only is our Etheric Body the primary controller of our Physical Body, but it is also our primary interface to the other energy bodies—the *Astral*, *Mental*, and *Causal Bodies*. One of the important places where these interconnections occur is the *central channel*—a line of energy that runs from the crown of the head down to the base of the torso. The central channel is also the primary region where interchanges between our Etheric Body and the greater etheric environment happen.

Most of you have probably heard of *chakras*—vortices of energy situated along the central channel. The chakras are important locations where energies are drawn into and out of the Etheric Body. For this reason, they have a big influence upon our health. There are seven primary chakras, each with its own functions, influences, and associated color. I describe them in detail in my book *Active Consciousness*,[1] but you can find out even more about them by researching online. The seven primary chakras are located near the perineum (red), the crown of the head (white), and along the front and back of the torso and the head— near the lower abdomen (orange), above the navel (yellow), the heart (green), throat (blue), and above and between the eyes (violet) (the so-called "third eye"). Teachings about the central channel and the chakras come primarily from India, and many meditative practices focus on them.

Of course, the architecture of the Etheric Body goes way beyond the central channel and the chakras. For instance, acupuncture and acupressure focus on a network of etheric energy channels called *meridians*, which run vertically throughout the body. Along these meridians are key energy exchange points—the targets of the acupuncturist's needles. While it may seem like these needles are used as some kind of physical intervention, what is really going on is that they tweak the etheric energy running along a meridian. After thousands of years of experience, practitioners have figured out how the meridians can be manipulated in order to heal at the etheric and, by extension, the physical level.

What happens to our Etheric Body after we die?

The Etheric and Physical Bodies need one another to exist. The Physical Body could not continue to operate if its Etheric Body were not running the show. But when our Physical Body dies, our Etheric Body eventually dissipates as well. Buddhists believe this process takes three days to occur and thus they delay burial until after that time. Rudolph Steiner taught that the information embedded within the Etheric Body (which includes traces of the brain's experiences) eventually drifts away and rejoins the collective etheric field.

But that's not the end of us!

After our physical death and the dissipation of our Etheric Body, our Astral, Mental, and Causal Bodies continue on. In fact, these even higher energy bodies are probably the most important factor that determines our sense of who we are. That's why people who have near death experiences report that they still feel like themselves after they "died," even when their Physical Body and brain stopped functioning.

Similarly, people who have out-of-body experiences (OBEs) report that they leave their Physical and Etheric Bodies behind as they travel around in their Astral, Mental, and Causal Bodies. While a person is having an OBE, their Etheric Body remains behind to "guard the physical fort," since the Physical Body can't function without it. An OBE'er then wanders off in Astral, Mental, and Causal form, but remains connected to their Physical and Etheric Bodies via an extended etheric energy cord (likely connected to the central channel). This cord emanates from their root chakra and enables them to return to their Physical Body once their travels are over. Amazing!

Now let's find out even more about these possibly immortal energetic components of our complete Selves.

CHAPTER 6

꒦

BEYOND THE
PHYSICAL AND ETHERIC

Even if you believe in some form of life after death, you may still assume that the dead are enlightened and all knowing. Not necessarily. Those who have had near-death experiences report that their sense of self remained essentially the same after they died. However, they also frequently come back with a deeper state of awareness and greater wisdom. After all, they have had proof that they are not merely their earthly Physical Body! They also report an experience of deep love and a knowingness that all of us are inherently interconnected and timeless.

How can this be? The explanation lies in the fact that our Astral, Mental, and Causal Bodies continue on, usually as a single unit, after our Physical Body dies and its etheric energy dissipates. (Note: sometimes I'll call this Astral-Mental-Causal unit the *Higher Body*.) In other words, after we die, we operate in a new, non-physical domain—one with its own operating principles. As I will discuss later on in this chapter, there is also evidence that this domain is common to *all* Higher Bodies between lives. Indeed, it may be our true home. If so, our incarnated physical lives may simply be relatively brief "learning" excursions that we participate in during our timeless existences. This notion is fundamental to the concept of *reincarnation*—that the life we are experiencing now is just one among many that have occurred and will occur in the future.

Most seers who have written about the higher energy bodies say largely the same things. The Astral Body is the locus of the emotional part of us. In modern psychological terminology, it may include (but is not limited to) the unconscious or subconscious mind. The teachings of Huna (based on Hawaiian shamanic wisdom) suggest that the Astral Body is also where all of our memories, inner feelings, and psychic abilities originate. In general, the emotions and sensitivity of the Astral Body are strongly influenced by experiences during childhood. While some aspects of our Astral Body may be discarded after a particular lifetime ends, there is still a memory of them retained for learning and growth during the period between incarnations.

The Mental Body, in contrast, is the prime controller of our rational, logical, planning, and calculating mind. Although this part of us is not very operational when we are young children, it becomes the "boss" of our Astral Body as we mature. That is why adults tend to suppress their emotional and intuitive Astral Body in subservience to the rational directives of their Mental Body. Rest assured, however—our inner astral feelings and experiences have not disappeared! Our Astral Body is *always* there, with its subterranean and unconscious emotional feelings and memories intact. And because it is the energy body most intimately connected with our Etheric and Physical Bodies, our Astral Body has a powerful role in creating and curing physical disease. I'll discuss this in detail later, especially in Chapter 16.

In contrast to the Astral and Mental Bodies, much less is written about the Causal Body. In most wisdom traditions, it is considered to be the wise self that always lies deep within us. That's why, after we die and the distracting physical aspects of our being depart, we tend to become more aware of it. In essence, the Causal Body is our personal piece of and link to the great universal love and source of All That Is—what we might call God or Great Spirit. In the terminology of the Course in

Miracles (an amazing teaching that is reputedly a channeled message from Jesus), the Causal Body is our piece of the Holy Spirit. It is also what enables us to be creators and manifestors—that is, beings created in "God's image." As I will discuss in Chapter 8, it is through our Causal Body that we are able to affect physical reality in unexpected ways.

At this point, you may be asking, "But isn't this all just a metaphor for something going on in my brain?" No. While your emotions, reasoning abilities, and wise insights do have correlates in your Physical Body, the *origins* of these functions are literally your Astral, Mental, and Causal Bodies—even if you are totally unaware of their existence.

Think of it this way. Just as the electronic signals firing in the circuitry of your television are not the origin of a TV program you watch—they are merely the result of the TV's mechanical operation after it receives an externally-generated signal—your physical brain and body may simply be biological structures that embody the directives of your Astral, Mental, and Causal Bodies. In other words, when you are physically alive, these higher energy bodies *inform* your Physical Body, with your Etheric Body playing a key role in the transmission process. After death, the Higher Body is still operating because it is intrinsically independent of the physical you. That's why near-death experiencers report having emotions and thoughts even when they are "outside" their bodies and brain-dead. They are still, essentially, themselves. They just don't have functioning Physical Bodies anymore.

In my view, one of the most accessible and useful sources of information about the higher energy bodies can be found in the wisdom of Huna[1]. According to Max Freedom Long, who developed Huna based on his encounters with Hawaiian shamans in the early 1900s, this knowledge originated somewhere in the Middle East and can be found encoded in the words of Jesus. It then migrated via the spiritual masters of Asia to make its way to Polynesia, eventually being brought to the Hawaiian Islands by the Tahitians about 1500 years ago. Others, however, say that the original spiritual masters of Hawaii were not

Tahitians, but rather, the mythical Menehune, people who reportedly lived on the islands long before the Tahitian migration. Wherever this knowledge originated, the Huna system is quite useful in practice. It describes the distinct functions, roles, and interrelationships between the Astral, Mental, and Causal Bodies and provides guidance on how to work with them.

The energy bodies, of course, go by different names in every culture around the world. Nevertheless, the content and methods of all these wisdom traditions are similar. They all stress that by understanding the functions of the higher energy bodies and by developing a relationship with them, we can achieve not only health and happiness, but also develop amazing abilities that enable us to affect the physical world and how reality unfolds. In other words, by deepening our understanding of and communication with these parts of our complete Selves, we can learn to better *live in synchrony*—both within and without. Let's begin your journey toward achieving this by taking a look at the Astral Body in greater detail.

THE ASTRAL BODY

In modern psychology, the Astral Body is usually equated with the subconscious or unconscious mind and is assumed to be a byproduct of a primitive part of our brain. Freud was certainly onto something when he asserted that this part of us plays a big role in determining our health and behavior. However, according to Huna and other wisdom traditions, the Astral Body encompasses much more than the conventional notion of the subconscious and goes way beyond the brain. It is actually *independent* of the Physical Body and has much more power than we normally give it credit for. Here are some of the important functions of the Astral Body according to Huna:

- **It is our most important link between our Higher Body and our Etheric Body**, and thus plays a vital role in our physical health. As we will learn in Part III, that is why so many self-healing systems focus on working with the Astral Body.

- **It stores all of our memories**. To our Astral Body, every moment of the past, including our birth, early childhood experiences, and perhaps even our past lives, are as near and present as if they were occurring at this moment.

- **It is the primary source of our inner emotions—how we really feel**.

- **It has no rational or reasoning ability**. Thus, when we plan, perform mathematical analyses, or focus on understanding something, the Astral Body is not involved; that is the purview of the Mental Body.

- **It is the primary locus of psychic abilities and our connections to the greater astral realm, which is a primary dwelling place of the Higher Bodies of both the living and the dead**. For example, when a genuine medium is communicating with someone who is dead, he or she is using their Astral Body to communicate with the Higher Body of the deceased person dwelling within the astral realm.

- **It is highly impressed and affected by what the Physical Body hears, sees, and feels—the physical senses**. These impressions can be a source of sustenance and healing (for example, seeing and smelling a beautiful flower or hearing blissful music) or of harm (watching a violent movie). Because the Astral Body has no reasoning ability or rational discernment (which are functions of the Mental Body), watching a horror movie or being told that something horrible is going to happen (like a doctor pronouncing your likely date of death) is taken as truth. Since the Astral Body can easily direct the Etheric Body and thereby affect the Physical Body, watching a horror movie or hearing someone predict your demise *can* invoke great physical terror and even death. But similarly, the Astral Body can also enable miraculous healing or physical protection from otherwise damaging activities.

Death and Out-of-Body Experiences (OBEs)

When we die, our Astral, Mental, and Causal Bodies tend to stay together. These comprise our complete Higher Body, which operates primarily in the astral realm—just as we are now operating primarily in the physical world with our Physical, Etheric, and Higher Bodies. Because we are still basically "ourselves" after we die (just without a Physical and Etheric Body), we may even, at least initially, feel like nothing has changed after we die.

However, in rare cases, the Astral Body can become detached from its corresponding Mental and Causal Bodies. This creates a ghost or poltergeist—an emotional Astral Body uncontrolled by a rational Mental Body or wise Causal Body. Shamans who are adept at operating at the astral level are sometimes called upon to help these wayward astral beings to move on and merge with their corresponding Mental and Causal Bodies. In some cases, they coax them to detach from the bodies of living people who have become invaded by them.

So, what do we find when we enter the astral realm? According to the teachings of the International Academy of Consciousness (IAC), this world is structured in a way that reflects the nature of the higher energy beings who inhabit it. The IAC cosmology was originally based on the teachings of two Brazilian psychic masters, Waldo Vieira and Francisco Candido Xavier. However, rather than simply echoing their teachings, the IAC focuses primarily on teaching students to experiment and discover this information for themselves. In particular, its workshops teach participants how to have an out-of-body experience (OBE), during which the Higher Body detaches from the Physical and Etheric Bodies. While it is possible for this to occur in a waking state, it is easier to achieve while dreaming, especially during lucid dreams. In Brazil, IAC centers foster these abilities and study the observations of OBE-ers. In essence, they are laboratories focused upon observing the astral world.[2]

In addition to teaching how to achieve an OBE, IAC workshops provide instructions on how to "see" the astral world with one's Astral Body while still fully grounded in the Physical Body. In one workshop I attended, I had the remarkable experience of seeing the face of a man superimposed upon the face of the female teacher. A couple of other people in the room saw the same thing and described the man's face in the same way. The "seeing" technique utilized breathing exercises in order to activate and intensify the sixth chakra, often called the "third eye," located in the forehead. I have always had some limited ability to see at the etheric level, so perhaps it wasn't surprising that I was one of the few people in the class who was successful during this exercise. The female teacher sat in front of us in a slightly darkened room, saying nothing but supposedly inviting astral beings to make themselves seen by superimposing themselves upon her face. I was shocked when I was able to distinctly see the face of a man obscuring her features. It was a convincing demonstration of the IAC message, especially when others reported seeing the same face.

According to the IAC, the astral realm is organized into levels or regions comprised of people who think and feel much the same way. Perhaps this is because it operates according to the principle of "like attracts like." For example, some regions are inhabited by people suffering from similar forms of negativity, greed, or criminality (various types of "hell"). Other regions are filled with more peaceful folk, perhaps with similar inclinations or interests (various kinds of "heaven"). The good news is that our existence within these regions can be fluid, so that a person doesn't remain stuck in one region forever if they undergo some kind of fundamental change. To get a good idea of the IAC conception of the afterlife, I recommend viewing the fascinating Brazilian movie *Nosso Lar* ("Our World"). The astral city depicted in this movie is based upon channeled information that Francisco Xavier received from the spirit of André Luiz, a prominent doctor who lived in Rio de Janeiro.

Perhaps an even more convincing account of the astral realm is described in the book *Journey of Souls* (and its follow-on books),[3] published by Michael Newton in the 1990s. Newton was a psychotherapist who specialized in therapeutic past life regression. At some point, however, he decided to develop techniques to take his patients even deeper and inquire about what happens after death and before reincarnation—that is, the period *between* lives. Remarkably, over the course of several years and 1000s of sessions, all of his patients reported essentially the same thing. Using illustrative session transcripts, *Journey of Souls* describes a world we all come from and enter back into, after death and until reincarnation.

Newton's underlying message is that our life between lives is all about reviewing what we learned during an incarnation and later, volunteering to engage in another incarnation in order to continue the learning process. According to his research, each of us chooses a particular period, location, and person to incarnate into. Nevertheless, the life we choose is not preordained. That is, while we *do* have a specific learning purpose or goal when we incarnate into a particular physical form, sometimes we succeed and sometimes we don't.

Newton also discovered that each of us has a cohort of astral beings that we study with during our life-between-lives. Often, some in our cohort volunteer to incarnate along with us into bodies that will play a key role in our learning as well as their own. Just before we incarnate, we are also given reminders that provide subtle prompts or clues to help us at critical moments. From my own life experience, I believe these prompts usually come in the form of significant synchronicities. In fact, both my husband Steve and I experienced remarkable synchronistic events during the time period that surrounded our first meeting in October 1981.

Journey of Souls had a profound impact on me and Steve when we read it in late 2020 and early 2021. It helped us to understand and accept that we had literally signed up for this life and the difficulties that we were experiencing during the COVID period. It became clear to us that the course of our lives over the preceding 35 years had led us to our ultimate decision to leave our home in California, travel the country, and find a new life elsewhere in the United States. When we hit the road in September 2021, we also made a conscious decision to notice unusual synchronicities that appeared along the way. Indeed, many things have continued to occur since that time that further convince us that we chose just the right place to ultimately land.

A Higher Dimensional World

In my view, the Astral Body and the astral realm likely exist in four-dimensional space. As I discussed in detail in my book *Active Consciousness,* being four-dimensional comes with many perks. If you are already adept at accessing your Astral Body, you likely already possess some of them: psychic abilities like remote-viewing ("seeing" things that are distant in time and space); inner-viewing (the ability to "see" inside three-dimensional objects, enabling powers like psychic medical diagnosis); and communication with the dead (mediumship).

There are many other amazing phenomena associated with our contact with the astral realm. For instance, there have been reports of communication with the dead via electronic devices.[4] Although it isn't easy for a non-physical astral being to interact directly with our three-dimensional physical world, it is not impossible. But even if direct contact cannot be made with us, a four-dimensional astral being can certainly visit and perceive our physical world. Some believe that such visitations are triggered when we focus upon a departed loved one.

That's how genuine mediums are able to make contact and facilitate communication between the deceased and their loved ones. If you have an interest in this subject, I recommend exploring the work of the Spiritualist Church,[5] which has branches all over the world, especially in the USA.

Another consequence of living in four spatial dimensions is the ability to create any reality that one expects or desires. The IAC reports that this is indeed the case in the astral realm. For example, they say that after someone dies but does not yet realize or understand what is going on, they tend to recreate the world they had been living in before. They may find themselves dwelling in a place much like their old home, perhaps embellished with things that they wished they had. Or they may create a heaven or hell in the form they were anticipating. That's why a Christian might meet Jesus, a Buddhist might see Buddha, and a Muslim might encounter Mohammed. Your afterlife meets your expectations!

Not surprisingly, the veil between the physical and astral worlds becomes especially thin around the time of death, as the Higher Body of the soon-to-be departed is separating from the physical. Many people experience visitations from their dead relatives at this time. My mother (who did not believe in the afterlife) had these kinds of "dreams" a few days before her death, reporting that dead relatives were waving to her and beckoning her.

Just after someone dies, the connection between their Higher Body and the physical world is still fairly strong. Because of this, surviving relatives often report psychic feelings or visions of their dead loved one trying to provide guidance and comfort. How is this possible? Through interactions between our Astral Bodies. When I was sorting through my mother's possessions a few days after she died, I said out loud, "How will I sell this condo, Mom?" I no longer had many connections to my hometown, which I had left nearly 40 years before. Just a minute later, as I was walking to my car, a neighbor came over and gave me the name of a real-estate agent. Coincidence, synchronicity, or a transmission from my mother in the astral realm?

Eventually, of course, most dead people realize that it is time for them to move on into their life between incarnations, knowing that they will likely reconnect with their loved ones after they too return to what may be our *true* home. Occasionally, however, the deceased have a hard time detaching from their physical life. Once again, shamans or mediums can be brought in to provide assistance and convince the dead to move on and focus upon their new "life-between-lives" in the astral realm.

Sleep, Lucid Dreams, and OBEs

Out-of-body experiences can occur while someone is awake or asleep. Since it is easier to achieve an OBE during sleep or just as you are falling asleep, the IAC focuses a great deal on the nature of the sleep process. They report that when a person is having an OBE, or even during normal sleep, their Astral, Mental, and Causal Bodies depart their Physical Body as a unit: the Higher Body. The Etheric Body, however, remains connected to the Physical Body, maintaining its functions. To make sure that the Higher Body is not "lost" during sleep or an OBE, an etheric energy cord tethers it to its corresponding Etheric Body, likely at the base of the central channel.

According to the observations of the IAC, during normal sleep, the Higher Body simply floats above the physical body, and standard dreams are simply a matter of the brain rehashing the day or other information. The Higher Body observes these dreams and records them as memories that are retained by the Astral Body.

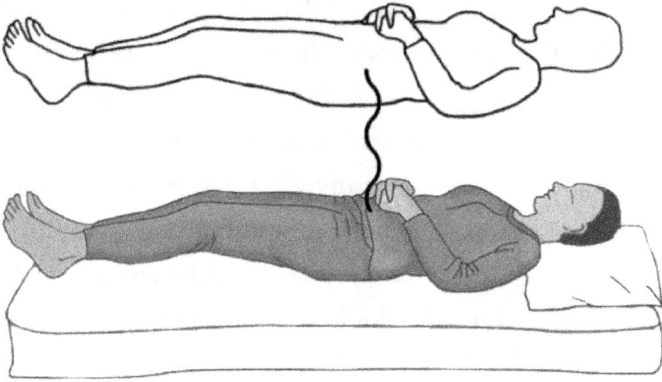

During an OBE, however, the Higher Body completely leaves the sleeping Physical Body behind. In some OBEs, it roams around the experiencer's familiar physical world. For example, it might explore a different country or visit a friend's house. In other OBEs, the Higher Body visits the astral realm itself. One sign that you have had an OBE is the memory of a "flying" dream. Those who can remember such OBEs sometimes report seeing other dreamers "swimming" or flapping their arms in an attempt to fly. An experienced OBE'er, however, knows that such machinations are not necessary at all. The Higher Body can roam around during an OBE in an erect posture and simply direct itself where it wants to go.

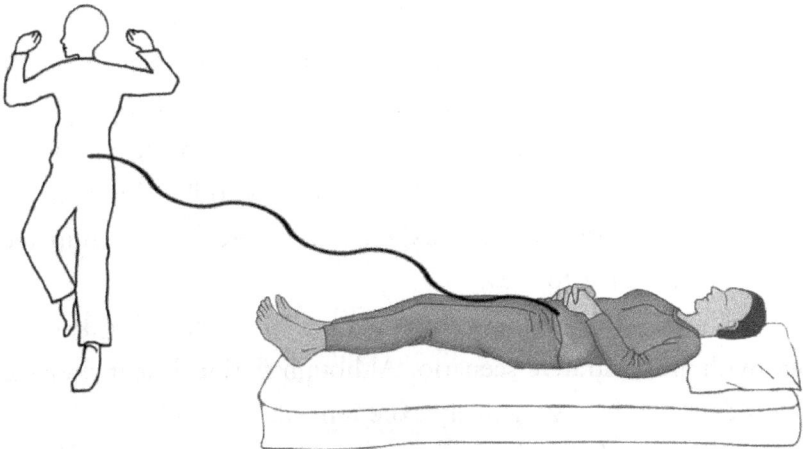

In some cases, the sleeping OBE'er can become "lucid"—that is, become cognizant that they are asleep and that their Higher Body has separated from their Physical Body. These experiences are quite memorable and are often recalled as being as vivid as normal physical life. I have had one such experience myself. I had already prepared a question to ask and, as a result, I believe I was given a glimpse of my death. During the lucid dream, I left my body and soared over San Francisco Bay, witnessing a future that looked nothing like it does today. True or not? Only time will tell.

I'm sure that almost all of you have had a flying dream. According to the IAC, all such dreams are OBEs, even if they are not lucid. If you would like to try to convert a flying dream into a lucid dream, train yourself (while you are awake) to say "I am dreaming" if you find yourself flying. If you can then achieve lucidity and maintain it, you might ask for some kind of information. Don't forget: the astral realm exists in four-dimensional space. From this vantage point, you are able to view your past and future, locate dead relatives, and visit other worlds entirely!

The IAC technique for triggering an OBE while you are awake involves rapidly running energy up and down the central channel. It's almost as if this process charges up your etheric tether to prepare you for "take off." The same breathing technique was a part of the astral "seeing" exercise I described earlier. The IAC workshops also describe various signs of an imminent OBE. These include an extremely heightened sense of sound, and feelings of physical rigidity or extreme heaviness (sometimes called sleep paralysis). Interestingly, shamanic teacher Hank Wesselman's books,[6] which describe his otherworldly visitations to the distant future, report that his experiences were always initiated by symptoms very similar to these.

To understand all of these ideas better, let's take a break now and engage with an illustrative scenario. Although fictional, it includes many elements that people have actually experienced.

CHAPTER 7

※

AN ASTRAL JOURNEY, PART I

I am running through a field as fast as I can, escaping from something, but what? All I know is that something is behind me and others are running too. Then a thought pops into my head: *Fly!* I look within and suddenly I know how to do it: jump and swim, with a breaststroke that grabs the air, air that feels as thick as water. Stroke, stroke, stroke, and I'm up! Flying through the air, I am safe.

Then another thought pops into awareness: *If I fly, I'm dreaming.* It's hard to stick with this, but I also know that I'm supposed to actually say it out loud: *If I fly, I'm dreaming.*

Suddenly everything around me becomes a bit clearer and visually sharper. The field is now empty, and there is no threat to be seen. With a light stroke, I glide gently through the air and the wind carries me. I can even smell the air. The sun is setting, just a glow in the distance. Beyond the forest to my left lies a distant mountain. *Why am I here? What's happening?* And suddenly I remember. *I must be having a lucid dream! Is this an out-of-body experience?*

I look down at my hands and then at my chest and legs. I am all there, but everything is shimmering and a bit fuzzy, tinged with an energetic glow. As I continue to stroke my arms through the air, I also notice a trail that's left behind me for a few moments, as if there's an energetic residue left behind. *Interesting!* I gaze at the tree line in the distance and notice a glistening silvery blue halo over it. It is enveloped in yellow, with arcs of energy reaching between the branches.

Below, I see a few scattered people hovering slightly above the field, swimming, gliding, or flapping in a daze. Swooping in for a better look, I notice that they too are enveloped in energy, each of them connected to a thin silvery white cord, like a kite string tethering them to some place in the distance. When I bend forward and look down between my own legs, I see that I, too, have a cord!

What's going on? What is all of this?

Suddenly I find myself in my darkened bedroom, floating near the ceiling. Below me lies my sleeping body with my "cord" connected to it. I also see that my body is enveloped in a soft silvery-blue energy and that this same energy runs along the cord attached to me.

At that very moment I realize that I'm not swimming anymore. *How am I just floating here, doing nothing to stay up?* I feel a tug, a shudder, pulling me back down. I resist! *No! I want to explore some more! Take me back to the field!* Instantly, I am transported back to the field. However, I can now just lift off or glide over the grass and trees in an upright position, simply by intending to do so.

Now I remember something about the "real world"—the world of my sleeping body back at home. Before turning off the light, I had suggested to myself that I would have a lucid dream. I've been reading books about the subject over the past few days and I had told myself that if I found myself flying, I would say, "If I fly, I'm dreaming." It worked!

I also remember that something else prompted me to try this. *What was it? Oh yes! My problems at work.* My boss, an older woman, is constantly blocking my progress at every step. She questions everything I do and nags me to do more. *Why doesn't she like me? I'm doing my best!*

Then a thought pops into my head. *Go see her.*

Suddenly, I find myself hovering above my city in the middle of the night. I feel drawn to a particular house in an older part of town. It is dark, like all the other houses, except for a dim light coming from a window on the second floor. I wonder who is in there and in an instant find myself hovering below the ceiling in that room. There I find my boss, kneeling beside the bed of a very old woman who is obviously sick and near death. My boss is gently stroking the woman's gray hair, talking to her in a soothing voice and occasionally giving her sips of water.

Slightly embarrassed by this intrusion into their privacy, I decide to return home. In the blink of an eye, I am back in the living room of my house, looking at the sleeping form of my housemate on the couch. *Passed out again, as usual!* I glide a bit closer to him and notice that, floating slightly above his body, is a shimmering energy-like replica of his form, connected not only by a single cord but by many threads of energy. Then I enter my other housemate's room and see the same phenomenon: twin forms, one physical and one energetic, connected by strands of silvery blue energy.

Suddenly I feel a tug, my own cord pulling me back. *What was it I read? How to stay lucid? Oh yes, twirl!* With all my might I pull myself into a spin and twirl right out of the house, like a whirling top soaring into the sky. And then I remember another thing I read about lucid dreams: I can ask a question. That, too, I had prepared in advance: *Why am I being blocked at work?*

I close my eyes for a moment. When I open them, I find that I have been transported back to my childhood hometown and everything looks like it did back then. *Why, there's my house!* My Dad's car is in the driveway. I descend to the ground and walk with trepidation toward the front door.

Suddenly, another being comes into view—a shimmering white form approaching me from down the street. I sense that this presence is kind and wise, and as it gets closer, I realize that it is a woman emanating a loving feeling towards me. Sensing that she has some kind of answer to my question, I ask again, *Why am I being blocked at work?*

The being takes my hand and transports me to the backyard of the house. And there I see myself! It's the younger me, about age eight, swinging on one of the swings next to my older sister. Tension fills me as I remember the rivalry and animosity I always felt between us. An angry and unhappy girl, my sister was always making my life miserable. Soon, my sister's friend emerges from the house and my sister gets off her swing. The two of them grab me and make me get off my swing so that my sister's friend can use it. Then, my sister pushes me to the ground, yelling "Get lost, loser!"

Now I remember: that feeling of frustration, always being blocked from what I wanted to do. I had to share my bedroom with my sister too, and it was torture. My childhood was permeated with the feeling that I could never get out from under her; that life just wasn't fair and I couldn't get ahead no matter what I did.

Then I feel the angelic being's presence again. She takes my hand, smiles knowingly, and gently hugs me. Suddenly, I get it. *Why do I feel blocked at work? It's my pattern from the past!*

With that realization, I feel a sudden whoosh. I open my eyes and I am back in my body, back in my bed. I've been asleep for only three hours. *Was all of this just a dream?*

CHAPTER 8

۶

I THINK *AND* I AM

THE MENTAL BODY

While it is true that some forms of mental processing take place inside the physical brain (and that these more shallow functions may potentially be simulated by artificial intelligence), the real locus of what we consider to be our mind is our energetic *Mental Body*. The Mental Body is where language, mathematics, and creative inspiration are all born.

Unlike the emotional and psychic astral realm, the mental realm is all about symbolism and meaning. It is where our significant dreams and their symbolic messages are developed. We remember these dreams when we awaken because they are stored as memories within our Astral Body. And if a shaman asks a question and then looks up into the sky for a "sign" or omen (like the appearance of a particular bird or weather pattern), it is because he or she understands that omens symbolize a response generated and transmitted from the mental realm. Indeed, the underlying mechanism of omens is likely due to the phenomenon of *synchronicity*—the co-occurrence in time and space of events related by meaning. I introduced this concept in Chapter 3 and will be discussing it in more detail later on in this chapter.

The Mental Body is also the source of our *will*—the part of us that applies discipline and helps us to get things done. Without our Mental Bodies, we humans would never have developed technology, agriculture,

71

medicine, art, or the wheel—and we would not have adapted so successfully to our everchanging Earth environment. In other words, this part of us is essential to our physical survival.

Needless to say, the Mental Body is the primary focus of today's developed societies, with their stress on schools, science, and culture. While a very young child operates primarily from their Physical and emotional Astral Bodies, by the time they reach the age of around eight or nine, their Mental Body comes into the foreground. Its dominance is then buttressed by the teachings we receive at school—reading, writing, and arithmetic. This also explains why a typical nine-year-old is obsessed with collecting things and memorizing facts. I remember how my son Izaak became fascinated by the American presidents at that age; he could recite them forwards or backwards in one breath! At parties, he would entertain our friends by asking for a number between one and forty-two and then regaling them with dozens of facts about the corresponding president.

Most people tend to be more highly developed in one of their bodies than the others. Some are very physically oriented, like superior athletes. Others tend to operate via their emotions or psychic intuitions. Then there are the academic types who "live in their heads." Just as a psychic may be very attuned emotionally and have a well-developed Astral Body (but may be less developed in the rational mental sphere), mentally-skilled academics who spend their lives pondering philosophy, science, and mathematics may be completely underdeveloped emotionally, psychically, or physically. Ideally, of course, we learn to develop in all spheres.

The Role of the Mental Body

One of the key jobs of the Mental Body is to guide the Astral Body. For example, it is our Mental Body that plans the day for us and gets us to finish our work before we indulge in our emotional desires. Chronic procrastinators, of course, may have an overbearing Astral Body that just won't listen! Nevertheless, the Astral Body is *usually* willing to accept a more subservient role and is faithful and eager to oblige. When the Mental Body wants to recall a memory, the Astral Body obeys and delivers its stored information for consideration. When the Mental Body suggests at bedtime that the Astral Body recall dreams for later decoding, our inner emotional self does its best to comply. And because the Astral Body is especially impressed by physical actions and sensations, if the Mental Body's directives are expressed as written instructions, are spoken out loud, or are accompanied by some sort of ceremony (even simply placing a pen and paper at bedside in order to record dreams), the results can be even better.

Because of its inherent subservience to the Mental Body, the Astral Body often decides to suppress its inner memories, desires, and emotions and hide them from conscious awareness—especially if it believes them to be unwelcome or unhelpful to the Mental Body. Unfortunately, the net effect of this strategy can be physical disease. Even though the Astral Body is withholding some memories and emotions from outward awareness and expression, it still holds them within itself. Since the Astral Body has an intimate relationship with and control over the Etheric Body (and thus the Physical Body), its subconscious feelings and memories may then express themselves in physical ways.

Chapter 16 will discuss two reasons for this pattern in detail. The medical revolutionary Dr. John Sarno[1] believed that the Astral Body's use of physical disease was a strategic way to *distract* the Mental Body. For example, by forcing the rational mind to focus on physical pain or some other troublesome physical symptom, the Astral Body may actually be trying to spare its boss, the Mental Body, from experiencing uncomfortable or unacceptable expression of its feelings. In contrast, I tend to believe that the Astral Body, though trying to suppress itself, is ultimately compelled to make its needs known in a physical way. Whatever the reason for this phenomenon, the Astral Body is not being malicious. It simply believes that physical problems are preferable to the Mental Body than outward expressions of anger, fear, or some other emotion.

Here's an example of this phenomenon. Suppose a woman is unhappy in her marriage but rationally knows that she must maintain a façade of happiness for her own or her children's safety. The net effect, however, is that she now develops chronic arthritis or back pain. These physical problems divert her conscious attention away from her deeper feelings of sadness—emotions that she might not consciously be aware of. Her physical symptoms might also help her to gain some much-needed attention or rest, or may provide her with an excuse not to engage with her spouse.

In truth, this kind of pattern is incredibly common. In fact, we all do it, in one way or another. Dr. Sarno believed that emotional suppression is the root cause of almost all disease, from the common cold to back pain to cancer. And that is why so many self-healing techniques focus on unearthing the true feelings of the Astral Body and developing an open relationship with it—to convince this part of us that the strategy of suppressing emotions and manifesting physical disease is no longer necessary or desirable. I will discuss this in more detail in Chapter 16.

Another unfortunate but common negative pattern of interaction between the Astral Body and Mental Body occurs when the rational power of the Mental Body is influenced by misguided astral emotions. Don't forget: although the Mental Body might be able to reason, its "data" generally comes from memories and perceptions stored within the Astral Body. This information might be quite prejudiced and misguided. It might have been influenced by media and propaganda, or biased by societal pressures, childhood memories, past traumas, and teachings from parents or other authority figures. Unfortunately, when a person enlists their rational mind to enact harmful actions based on this kind of information, wars and other kinds of violence can result.

Another example of this phenomenon is when a skilled scientist becomes coerced by fear or convinced by propaganda or financial greed to use their mind to develop harmful technology. If they are motivated by fear, they may be mentally aware that their actions are harmful. But if they are motivated by greed or anger, they may mentally rationalize their actions and create what G.I. Gurdjieff called "buffers," which shield them from thinking about the consequences of their actions.

The bottom line is that when someone uses their Mental Body to create harmful outcomes, they have become disconnected from the innate wisdom and guidance of their Causal Body. A terrorist may believe it is "logical" to use their mental skill to harm others because it aligns with what they have been taught or accepted emotionally. But they have also lost their connection to a deeper and more loving part of themselves. An extreme example of this is an insane dictator like Hitler or Stalin. Because these men's sick and damaged Astral Bodies and willful Mental Bodies were especially good at manipulating others, they were able to wield tremendous power through the use of fear and the impact of their words. Luckily, our Causal Bodies ultimately have even more intrinsic power.

THE CAUSAL BODY

Many people refer to their inner self as their "soul." Others talk about their "spirit." But what's the difference? In my view, these terms likely refer to different components of our complete energy body. I believe that the "soul" consists of our Astral and Mental Bodies, whereas the "spirit" is our Causal Body or what might be called the High Self or our piece of the Holy Spirit.

Our Causal Body is the part of us that connects us to *all that is*—the universal and infinite field of energy that some people call God, Brahman, or Great Spirit. In essence, it is our little piece of Source. It might seem hidden or remain unacknowledged by us, but it is an essential part of who we are and what we are capable of. And it is always within us and available to provide its wise love and guidance—if we only learn to interact with and pay attention to it.

When we earnestly pray, for instance, we are actually communicating with our Causal Body. As visionary Neville Goddard[2] said, "Christ" is not a person who lived 2000 years ago, but instead is something that can be found within each one of us. In his view, if we "access God through Christ," it means we are accessing the whole through our piece of the whole—our Causal Body. It is this aspect of our being that an enlightened guru is referring to when he or she says "I Am That" or "I AM." Also recall that God is described in the Bible with almost the same words: "I Am That I Am."

Unlike our emotional Astral Body and rational Mental Body, our Causal Body is our deepest source of inner wisdom and knowing. It is loving, blissful, and joyful. If you believe that your Causal Body is telling you negative and hurtful things about yourself or others, think again! That's your Astral Body talking.

Our Causal Body is also our conduit to the larger source of creation. It's what makes us "beings created in God's image." That is, it gives us the ability to manifest and create. Perhaps that's why it's called the *Causal* Body. Manifestation techniques like the one described in my book *Active Consciousness*[3] or the Huna technique I'll describe in Chapter 9 are all based on developing a connection with this part of ourselves. By communicating with it, we are able to receive guidance that helps us to choose or create unlikely pathways into the future—from getting a perfect parking spot to curing ourselves of supposedly "incurable" diseases.

One mistake that many seekers make is believing that they can forget all about their Astral and Mental Bodies and simply hook up directly to their Causal Body. While establishing such a connection is always a great thing to do, the fact remains that our Astral Body and Mental Body are still there and won't just "go away." There may be a few rare people who experience spontaneous enlightenment, evolve their Astral and Mental Bodies in seconds, and manage to remain primarily in a state of contact with their Causal Body from that moment forward. But most of us can't perform this kind of "spiritual bypass."

The fact is, we are here on planet Earth with our Physical, Etheric, Astral, and Mental Bodies for a reason. I believe it's to learn lessons from our life experiences—both the good ones and the bad ones. That's why the process of spiritual evolution for most people is all about engaging in this learning process and especially, about working to evolve their Astral Body.

So how do we communicate with our Causal Body?

The most common technique is meditation. By quieting our emotions and thoughts and just being in the Now, we can achieve a more peaceful state and sometimes receive guidance from within. I call these whispers from our "still small voice within," *messages.*

But how can we distinguish a true message from more common wishful thoughts and feelings? First, remember that your Causal Body is a part of you. So it *will* communicate with you through your thoughts (your Mental Body), emotions (Astral Body), and sensations (your Physical and Etheric Bodies). Nevertheless, genuine messages from the Causal Body do have a different quality to them than everyday thoughts, feelings, and sensations. Usually, they occur spontaneously and feel as though they've arrived from outside yourself. They are also typically accompanied by feelings of inner knowing and joy. They simply don't have the same quality as self-delusional or wishful thinking. Of course, we all delude ourselves at times, even during meditation. But with experience, you can begin to discern the difference.

Another way the higher energy realms communicate with us is through *synchronicities*. I've already discussed this phenomenon briefly and its discovery by psychiatrist Carl Jung in the early 1900s.[4] This is how it happened. One of Jung's patients was recounting her dream about a golden scarab beetle when Jung heard a rapping on the window. When he opened it, a rose chafer beetle—the insect most similar to a scarab in his region—flew into the room. Jung quickly put two and two together. He realized that the mythological meaning of the scarab—an ancient Egyptian symbol for rebirth—was highly pertinent to his patient's problems. This synchronistically resulted in her dream. And her recounting of the dream in the clinic synchronistically caused the insect to appear at the window in waking life.

I believe that the appearance of various objects, people, occurrences, or significant dreams in our lives is a key way in which our higher energy bodies (as well as other beings operating in the astral, mental, and causal realms) communicate with us. An object may appear in an important dream because it meaningfully *symbolizes* the message of the dream. The unusual appearance of a certain animal in waking life may likewise be transmitting a symbolic message. When you think of a long-lost friend and they call you an hour later, it might be because your psychic Astral Body had a premonition. Alternatively, it might be a synchronicity coordinated by both your and your friend's Causal Bodies in order to bring you together for some important reason.

That's why I like to be on the alert for synchronicities. Some of them might be simple coincidences. Others might be the higher energy fields of meaning causing a "line up" between meaningfully related things. And some might be important messages from the causal realm whose purpose is to lead you in a certain direction. If you think back on your life, you may discover that significant turning points in your life were accompanied by synchronicities. I wrote about a few such experiences in my book *Active Consciousness*. And as I will discuss in the next chapter, synchronicities are also one of the key mechanisms behind the power of manifestation techniques.

Finally, let's not forget the name of this book—*Living in Synchrony*. When we line up with all of our complete beings, we activate the full powers of our Physical, Etheric, Astral, Mental, and Causal Bodies. This enables us to not only achieve health, but also to "sync up" with the greater energy realms we are a part of. When we do, seemingly miraculous synchronicities truly do happen!

CHAPTER 9

OPENING THE DOOR OF CREATION

In the last chapter, I discussed how the Causal Body is our link to All That Is—God, Great Spirit, the source of all creation. Because of this, it is also the source of our own ability to manifest and create. It is the Causal Body that enables us to choose more beneficial pathways into the future—the ones that bring us to a specific desired goal. In my book *Active Consciousness*, I call this process *manifestation*. Our Causal Body may also have the power to affect the likelihood that certain possible futures—even seemingly impossible ones—emerge into being. That is what I call the power of *creation*.

As an example of manifestation, the Causal Body might guide us to drive in a particular way—choosing the right route at the right time—so that we arrive at an important event on time or avoid a horrible accident. Or it might "whisper" things to us that help coordinate external events and guide us so that we get the perfect job or meet our life partner. In contrast, it is our ability to *create* that could enable our body to heal itself in unexpected or even "impossible" ways.

So how can we tap into these abilities more effectively?

Many books have been written about this topic and they all contain similar advice and steps to take. My book *Active Consciousness* is one of them, and in it, I also try to explain how they might actually work. In my view, our higher energy bodies—our Astral, Mental, and Causal Bodies—have access to higher dimensional space. Because our current physical life in three dimensions is just one of an infinite number of possible trajectories through these higher spatial dimensions, our higher-energy-bodies' access to these more expanded realms enables them to guide us through our limited three-dimensional reality more expertly.

Probably one of the simplest techniques for manifestation and creation is the Ha Ritual utilized in Huna. The rest of this chapter will describe it in detail. I was unaware of Huna and the Ha Ritual when I wrote *Active Consciousness*. If I had been, I would have added a bit more to the four steps I described in that book, because they left out a couple of useful details. Other manifestation methods tend to leave these steps out too. Still, the overall pattern is the same. Now that you understand more about the nature and powers of the Astral, Mental, and Causal Bodies, the logic of the Ha Ritual will make sense to you.

The Ha Ritual

The overarching process of the ritual begins by formulating the desired goal intention using the rational powers of the Mental Body. The next step is to enlist the all-important power of the Astral Body to gather energy (what Huna calls *mana*) in the Etheric as well as in the Astral, Mental, and Causal Bodies. Next it activates the emotional desire to make contact with the Causal Body and enlists its help in achieving the goal intention. If all goes well, we then simply need to let go and trust that the intended goal will be brought about. One of the ways this can happen is that the Causal Body "rains down" information that guides us. This may take the form of synchronicities, intuitions, omens, dreams, and the like. It is up to us to pay attention to this information and take action.

Note that the Astral Body plays perhaps the most important role in the manifestation and creation process. How so? First, it is the Astral Body that energizes the connection (perhaps via the central channel) running from the Etheric Body to the Causal Body. It then transmits the goal intention (formulated by the Mental Body) and releases it to the Causal Body.

But perhaps the most important role of the Astral Body in this process is the one omitted from most manifestation techniques: its required willingness to participate. If your subconscious inner emotions and beliefs do not really want a goal to be realized, your Astral Body will not truly cooperate, even if you go through the steps of the ritual. For instance, if you consciously think you want to meet your ideal mate or become financially successful, but at the same time, subconsciously believe you don't deserve a good relationship or that money is evil, it is unlikely you will succeed in your manifestation efforts. Similarly, if you consciously want to be healed of a disease but subconsciously want to hold on to it—for a variety of possible reasons—then your efforts to create healing will not be as effective.

That is why engagement with your Astral Body is so critical. After all, it is the part of your overall Higher Body that is most intimately connected to your Physical Body and Etheric Body, and thus exerts the most control over your physical health. Put all of this together and you can understand why so many self-healing techniques and Huna itself work hard to uncover the hidden beliefs, fears, anger, resentments, and guilt hiding within all of us that are holding us back.

Now let's go through the steps of the ritual in more detail.

1. Create a statement expressing your goal intention and write it down on a piece of paper. It is important that it be worded in the present tense, as if it is already true, not as something that you want to occur in the future. For instance, "I have a wonderful and fulfilling relationship with a life partner" is a good

formulation, but "I *want* to have a wonderful and fulfilling relationship" is not. Why? Because the second formulation implicitly connects you to the feeling that you *don't* have a good relationship. Other examples of effective goal statements are: "I love my job and everyone I work with and enjoy going to work each day," "I experience optimal health and freedom in my body and in my spirit," and "My body is vigorous and flexible."

2. Create a little shrine or area where you place this statement. I like to incorporate a candle and meaningful stones and objects I have gathered. Remember that your Astral Body is very impressed by these physical objects and actions, so your shrine and written statement and the steps of the Ha Ritual make up a critical part of enlisting its cooperation. In other words, *thinking is not enough; you have to **do** something.* To better engage my own Astral Body, I have also created a written statement that I use to ask for its cooperation. Your own statement might include words that apologize for ignoring its feelings and needs, express love for it, and promise to be more caring in the future, listening to its wishes and deep-seated emotions more fully.

3. Now it's time to begin. Settle into your body using whatever meditative technique you prefer. Personally, I focus on the sensations in my feet, seat, and back. For more guidance on meditation, check out the exercises I provide in *Active Consciousness*.

    Once you feel present and centered, it's time to gather *mana*, the Hawaiian word for energy. I believe that mana is the basic substrate of all the energy bodies, including the Etheric Body. When you gather mana, you are essentially activating your central channel and your link to the Higher Body. All you need to do is a simple breathing exercise: breathe in for a count of four, hold your breath for a count of four, breathe out for a count of four, and then remain empty for a count of four, all while holding the intention of gathering mana within you.

Here is how I like to perform this part of the Ha Ritual:

a. Repeat the four-step breathing process four times.
b. Ask (out loud) for the cooperation of your Astral Body, Mental Body, and Causal Body.
c. Repeat the breathing process again four times.
d. Read (out loud) your statement of love to your Astral Body.
e. Perform the breathing process again four more times.
   At this point you should feel very energized, in the moment, joyful, and connected to your entire being. In essence, you have entered into what I call in *Active Consciousness* the state of **NOW+**.

4. It's time to invoke your goal intention. Repeat it (out loud) four times. Each time, say it slowly, clearly, and try to fully feel that the statement is true, without doubt. It is important that you try to truly *be* in the intended goal state. (This is what I call in *Active Consciousness*, **PURE GOAL**.)

5. You are now ready to send your prayer up to your Causal Body along the energy channel you energized with mana. It is sent from your Astral Body up to your Causal Body. Slowly raise both hands upward over your head and send the prayer upward, saying the words, "The prayer has flown. So be it."

6. The ritual is now complete. Blow out your candle and dismantle your shrine in a state of calm knowing that all will be brought to you at the right time and in the right way.

Now it's time to engage in the last two steps I describe in *Active Consciousness*: **LET GO** and **CHOOSE JOY**. "Letting Go" means avoiding doubt (which creates blockages in the Astral Body) and trusting in the process—hence the statement, "The prayer has flown. So be it." It is also helpful to engage earnestly with your Astral Body on a regular basis and uncover any subconscious blocks to achieving your goal. Many of the tools and modalities I describe in Chapter 16 will help you to do this.

In the coming days and weeks, you must now stay alert for moments in which guidance is provided to you. Are you noticing synchronicities that occur each day? Do you record your dreams and try to decode them? Are you alert for sudden intuitions and inspirations? In Huna, this guidance is likened to "mana raining down." Indeed, the Bible uses the same term, "manna," for the "food" that rained down upon the Children of Israel as they wandered through the desert. Coincidence? I don't think so. After all, this was their journey to redemption and the achievement of their ultimate goal, the Promised Land.

Finally, when you make decisions, **CHOOSE JOY**. This means that you should use your internal sense of joy to accurately assess what's happening and to determine which actions to take. It can be helpful to meditate in order to access this inner sensation, realizing that the options that feel most joyful are most likely the right ones.

Before I conclude this chapter, I thought it would be useful to mention the work of three teachers whose books have inspired my own efforts at manifestation and creation. The first, of course, is the work of Max Freedom Long, the creator of Huna. He also describes how Huna is related to information in the New and Old Testaments.[1] Two other writers who have written about how the process of manifestation is encoded in biblical teachings are Florence Scovel Shinn (check out her well-known book from the 1920s, *The Game of Life and How to Play It)*[2] and visionary writer Neville Goddard.[3] A more contemporary writer, Tosha Silver, cites Shinn as the key inspiration for her own work and writing.[4]

Speaking of odd "coincidences," it turns out that Tosha Silver and I went to summer camp together nearly 50 years ago (when her name was Nancy Silver). I only found out about her work when a friend of mine introduced me to her brother. Upon learning about my own books, he told me about his "way out sister" who now goes by the name Tosha. Small world. Or a synchronicity?

Let's continue now with the scenario I began in Chapter 7.

CHAPTER 10

꙳

AN ASTRAL JOURNEY, PART II

I look at the clock. It's only 2am. As I get up to go to the bathroom, I recall some things I've read about manifestation and shamanic prayer rituals. *Maybe now is the time to try them out?*

Sitting on the edge of my bed, I reflect on my lucid dream and realize that it verifies many of the things I've read about. There *is* an energy body surrounding my physical body. I also have some kind of energy body double that detaches and moves around while I sleep, along with an energy cord that connects it back to my physical body. Thinking more about my dream, I realize that I have always felt a bit tense and frustrated, like I'm being blocked. *Maybe it all began with my sister?*

Suddenly I recall reading something about removing negative feelings; cutting them off in some way. I close my eyes and imagine that there are cords of energy penetrating my solar plexus, just above my navel, that link me to my sister. *Yes, that's where they seem to be!* There also seem to be cords that connect me to my sister from my throat and chest area. I start sweeping my hands in front of these areas, cutting and wiping away the cords, like sweeping away old cobwebs. Oddly, I feel a sense of relief. *I'll have to remember this the next time I feel frustrated at work!*

That reminds me of something else. *OK, now I have to do some kind of ritual to improve things at work.* In my closet I find an old, beautiful candle that my grandmother gave to me for my birthday. I reflect with a smile on what a sweet soul my Granny was. She really had a knowing spirit. I write something down about what I want, but as if I already had it.

"I am free, supported, and empowered at work, and I have wonderful relationships with my colleagues."

Wow! That feels good.

I place the candle on my dresser, along with my prayer message and a special stone I found on the beach to add that extra touch. Then I sit on the edge of my bed and try to enact the manifestation ritual I read about.

First I breathe in to a count of four. Then I hold it for four counts. Then I breathe out to a count of four. And then I remain empty for four counts. *That's simple!* I do it four times, each time imagining that I am bringing more energy into my body. *Maybe that's what charges up that silvery blue energy and the cord?* Now, I move on to the next step of the ritual and talk out loud to myself, using the following words:

"I call upon my feeling Astral Body, my thinking Mental Body, and my wise Causal Body to join together with me in my prayer."

I wonder: do these bodies have something to do with the energy body that I inhabited during my out-of-body lucid dream experience? And who was that angelic girl, anyway?

I decide to bring in more energy, with four more breathing cycles. *That feels right.* I feel a peaceful energy permeating me, and a grounded, knowing feeling. *Now must be the time for the prayer.* I repeat it four times, each time with deeper feeling and conviction, feeling its truth. It *is* true!

"I am free, supported, and empowered at work, and have wonderful relationships with my colleagues."

Now with a sweep of my hands into the air, I send the prayer up to my Causal Body, concluding with the statement, "The prayer has flown. So be it!"

I guess that's it! Now I'm just supposed to wait and trust, 'Just flow' as they say. Well, we'll see! I blow out the candle, get back into bed, and fall asleep quickly.

The next day I oversleep and get into work a bit late. *Oh wow, not a great way to begin my new empowerment on the job!* As I park my car in the lot, I notice something a bit odd. There are hardly any cars there! What's going on? I walk up to the front door of the building and see a sign posted. "The power has gone out. Work is cancelled for today. Report as usual tomorrow."

Lucky break! What's the chance of that? So what should I do? A whole day to myself! I walk across the street to the coffee shop and order a latte and a celebratory chocolate muffin. As I leisurely sip my coffee and nibble on my treat, I find a copy of my favorite newspaper abandoned on a table nearby. *This is the life!*

After an hour, as I skim the movie section of the paper, I notice that a nearby theater is showing a movie I've always wanted to see. Most theaters don't open until late in the afternoon, but this one has a show at 11am. *Sounds great! I have enough time to get there.* As I enter the slightly darkened and mostly empty theater, I am surprised to see my boss sitting there. *Hm. Should I go hide and sit somewhere where she won't notice me? No, that doesn't feel right. This feels like an opportunity...*

I walk up to my boss, who is equally surprised to see me. We have a few minutes before the movie starts, so we awkwardly start talking about the power outage at work. Then, surprisingly, my boss says, "Truthfully, I'm really relieved that work was cancelled today. I'm exhausted. I was up all night nursing my mom. I think she might die in the next few weeks. This movie is a real treat for me, a little get away."

Wow! My dream was true! What I saw was actually happening!

I commiserate with my boss, telling her about the death of my own mother a couple of years ago. I can tell that a new bond has now formed between us. After the movie, she says that she should get back home to her mother and I head out for a late lunch at a nearby diner.

Sitting at lunch, as I reflect on the amazing events of the past day, I am filled with a feeling of gratitude. *Isn't life amazing? Yesterday, I was angry and had a huge chip on my shoulder. Today I feel as light as a feather! And yes, my sister was a total pain, a bully. But it did teach me a thing or two about how to endure, how to keep pushing. Besides, the bullies of this world seem pretty unhappy inside. Maybe being a bully feels even worse than being their victim.*

With these thoughts, I notice a bit of that old frustration welling up inside me, so I sweep my hand in front of me and cut those cobwebs from the past. I look out the window at the beautiful day. With a smile, I realize that I am actually looking forward to going to work tomorrow and seeing my boss. *Maybe I'll even ask her to have lunch with me!*

CHAPTER 11

)ᴎ

A GREATER COSMOLOGY

At this point, I've painted a detailed cosmology that describes who and what we are. It includes the nature of our Physical and energetic Etheric and Higher Bodies, what happens when we have an out-of-body experience, and a bit about the nature of the afterlife. In this chapter, I will add in a few more interesting details. While this information isn't critical to understanding the rest of the book, I find it fascinating—so I thought you might too. At the very least, it will give you food for thought.

VISUALIZING WHAT WE ARE

From the standpoint of those who can see the human aura, we appear much like what was depicted in the figure in Chapter 5—a Physical Body at the dense center of our being, surrounded and interpenetrated by the layers of the Etheric, Astral, Mental, and Causal Bodies. But perhaps this is simply what we humans are *able* to see when we are locked into three-dimensional physical form. Our view or perspective might be limited by the context in which we are living.

In contrast, those who have had a near-death experience say that leaving their Physical Body feels like they are shedding a constrictive shell. It's almost as if being incarnated into a three-dimensional form is a kind of imprisonment—a throttling down of our expansive higher dimensional fullness into a more limited 3D form. After death, NDErs report that they feel liberated from this constriction and, instead, feel a sensation of lightness, relief, and freedom. Moreover, when they then decide to return to their Physical Bodies, they feel reluctance about being confined to a physical shell once again.

Another piece of information to consider is what wisdom teachers like Gurdjieff and Steiner, as well as the teachings of the IAC, say about the human physical/energy structure. They claim that if we *do* manage to evolve sufficiently (after several lifetimes of physical incarnation) and no longer need to incarnate again, we become long-term Astral-Mental-Causal beings living in the Astral World. If we evolve even further, we may then shed our Astral Body and become Mental-Causal beings living in the Mental World. Finally, our ultimate destination may be to evolve into purely Causal beings, living at one with All That Is in the Godly realm. If that is true, the process of evolution may be more akin to one of shedding, and the figure below may represent a more accurate picture of what's going on.

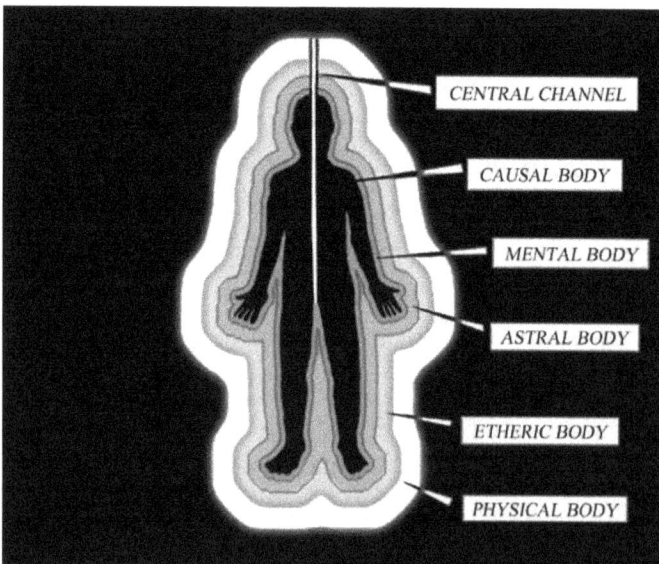

In this visualization, the Physical Body is depicted as a white outer shell built upon an Etheric Body. Within are the Astral, Mental, and Causal Bodies that comprise who we really are inside—our Higher Body. When we are alive, the powers of our Higher Body are transmitted to our Etheric Body and then, by extension to the Physical Body. Once our Physical Body dies, however, our physical shell is shed much as a snake sheds its skin. According to Buddhist teachings, the Etheric Body then gradually dissipates. At this point, we become an Astral-Mental-Causal energy being (our Higher Body), with our Astral Body as our outer "shell." We enter a realm that is primarily astral (just as we are now living in the physical realm in Physical Bodies). But within, we still have access to our rational Mental Body and wise Causal body.

ANIMALS, ELEMENTALS, AND DEVAS

So what about animals? Plants? Minerals? Do they have Etheric, Astral, Mental, and Causal Bodies too?

Both Gurdjieff and Steiner said that all living beings and even rocks and minerals have an Etheric Body. I tend to think of the etheric realm as the energy aspect of physical existence, much like an electromagnetic field that surrounds all physical things. That's why our Etheric Body slowly dissipates after death.

However, there is evidence that most living things have higher energy bodies too. For example, many people experience the Astral Bodies of their deceased pets when they dream or have an out-of-body experience. Mediums who can communicate with the astral realm also report animal encounters. Animals are even believed to reincarnate. But what about plants? People who are able to communicate with trees and other forms of vegetation report that they are able to pick up emotions and even the thoughts of these living beings. My hypothesis is that all living beings possess at least an Astral Body.

This brings us to an intriguing question. Are there energy beings who *cannot* possess physical form? People from almost all cultures describe encounters and communication with such mythical creatures. First, consider the so-called *elementals*. These beings often appear in books like the *Hobbit* and *Lord of the Rings*. They include faeries, elves, goblins, gnomes, leprechauns, and mermaids. Elementals are usually organized into groupings that correspond to the "four elements"—earth, air, fire, and water. For example, a leprechaun is an earth elemental, as are many of the other elementals that humans reportedly encounter. I have found the nonfictional work of Tanis Helliwell, who describes her experiences with leprechauns,[1] to be especially interesting.

Most writings about elementals assert that their primary role is to nurture the growth and maintenance of the physical world. For example, earth elementals help trees and flowers to grow, water elementals help cleanse the seas and deal with other forms of precipitation, air elementals help control atmospheric conditions, and fire elementals work with various forms of energy, like fire and radiation. Perhaps when people communicate with a plant or try to affect the weather, they are actually doing so with the help of elementals. Certainly, skilled shamans who work within the various energy realms have contact with these beings.

What about *devas*? According to some sources I have read, devas are essentially advanced or evolved elementals who control much larger spheres of influence. For example, a deva's domain might be an entire forest or a city. At the pinnacle is our planetary deva—a being we call Gaia.

In my opinion, elementals are strictly astral beings without Mental or Causal Bodies. This jibes with what Tanis Helliwell writes about them. As she points out, leprechauns are extremely emotional but not rational. According to Helliwell, however, advanced leprechauns are now trying to evolve and develop their mind (that is, develop a Mental Body) and to also gain the ability to manifest (develop a Causal Body). She also suggests that the realm of the elementals is four-dimensional. Because humans also possess a four-dimensional Astral Body, people who are psychic (that is, have a good connection to the astral realm) are often able to see elementals. In fact, Helliwell leads workshops to help people develop this skill.

Other informative books about elementals and devas include writings about places like Findhorn[2] and Perelandra.[3] These amazing communities are made up of people who engage with elementals in order to understand what nutrients plants need and want, as well as their desired arrangement. Using this knowledge, they have been able to grow unusually large and exotic plants—even tropical plants—in the barren northern soils of Scotland.

OVERSOULS AND ANGELIC BEINGS

And what about even higher energy beings—those who reside primarily in the mental and causal realms?

If you watch the movie *Nosso Lar*,[4] which depicts the cosmology of the IAC, you will notice that at critical junctures in the film, a being of light appears within the astral realm who guides people after they die in the physical world. Light beings also periodically appear and guide the main character of the movie, as he shifts his state of consciousness from one of despair and darkness to one of hope. I believe such light beings are *angels*—mental or possibly even causal beings. While astral beings help to shepherd us after we die and sometimes whisper guidance or create useful synchronicities for us during our physical lives, angels have even more power and wisdom to offer.

More evidence for the existence of astral, mental, and causal beings is found in the *Seth Teachings*, channeled by Jane Roberts from the 1960s until her death in 1984.[5] In them, Seth describes a particular kind of being called an *oversoul*. Oversouls have many roles, including guiding us during the death and reincarnation process and helping us to figure out what we need to accomplish when we reincarnate. A hierarchy of oversouls is also described by Seth, with some oversouls being the "bosses" of others. Interestingly, such beings are also described in the life-between-lives material of Michael Newton. In fact, their description is quite specific and detailed; they possess different colored energies depending on their level of achieved evolution and wisdom. Are these oversouls and over-oversouls astral, mental, and causal beings?

Finally, what about so-called "aliens"? Are they physical beings from other worlds like our own who have mastered interstellar travel? Or are some of them actually higher energy beings like angels and oversouls? Perhaps one day we will find out.

In the meantime, let's conclude Part II by considering the ultimate question.

CHAPTER 12

꒜

THE PURPOSE OF LIFE

What's the point of all this anyway? Why are we here on planet Earth? And what should our purpose or goal be while we're here?

In my view and in the view of many others, the reason why we repeatedly incarnate into physical form is to learn and evolve into beings possessing greater wisdom. At the most fundamental level, we are each a piece or an extension of God or Source. And because we are created in God's image, we can serve to expand all of creation through our own creations and experiences. By learning and evolving, we are enabled to add even more to that greater whole.

But why do we need to incarnate into physical form in order to do so? Let's consider the reincarnation process in more detail.

When we exist between lives within the astral world, we are higher dimensional and can thus create whatever we imagine or desire. If our development and awareness is limited, our creations will be similarly limited and will reflect our state of being. For example, someone who is emotionally mired in anger, hatred, greed, and self-loathing, will likely end up in an astral realm populated by people with similar tendencies (a so-called "hell"). But if someone's nature is generally loving and kind, their astral sojourn will likely be quite pleasant, though perhaps limited in other ways. Happily, physical incarnation offers us an opportunity to *change and learn*—that is, to fundamentally shift. How so?

Think about it. If you are able to create any object or situation just by thinking about it, you would likely never be motivated to work hard or learn anything. In contrast, when you are subjected to the slow and painstaking nature of physical life, you become deeply impressed by cause and effect—not just the effects of your own actions, emotions, and thoughts, but those of others as well. Because of this, physical incarnation can teach us some very important lessons—about love, relationships, art, nature, poverty, illness, unhappiness, loneliness, and violence.

In other words, physical incarnation is a rough but effective training ground. You may get mired in it all and not make much headway, or you might transcend, learn, and possibly even change your state for the better—even within a single lifetime. Each new incarnation, precisely designed and selected by us (a process described in detail in the books by Michael Newton), provides a new opportunity to learn and grow. Whether we decide to do so or not is up to us. Luckily, there is a silver lining. Many teachers claim that at the very least, we do not *de*-volve— that is, unlearn previous levels of awareness. So, we do retain what we have already learned.

Of course, that doesn't mean each lifetime becomes easier and easier. For example, if you've just led a life of luxury or excellent health, you may then decide to incarnate into poverty or illness in order to learn new lessons. The fact that we (at least initially) forget our astral and former physical lives after incarnation is a part of this process. By fully experiencing our childhoods and life experiences on a clean slate, we are primed to fully learn within the context of a chosen incarnated form— including sorrows that would not be experienced in the same way if we retained full knowledge of past incarnations or our life between lives. Note as well that the incarnation process may not be co-linear with Earth time. Thus, you might decide to incarnate into the distant past or the distant future—perhaps even onto an entirely different planet as an entirely different kind of being!

Here's another interesting question to ponder. *What exactly is the nature of the incarnational learning process?* The writings of Neville Goddard provide some insight.[1] Like many teachers in the area of manifestation or New Thought, Goddard stressed that our own consciousness, coupled with that of the rest of humanity, *creates* our experienced reality. In other words, *our life experience can be used as a powerful feedback mechanism that reflects back to us our inner state.* If you want to understand your current state of being, check out what's happening in your life.

From this standpoint, we are *always* living in synchrony—with our current inner state. For example, if you have low self-esteem, you will tend to experience events that reflect that state and, as a result, you may find yourself surrounded by others who have low self-esteem or who perpetuate your self-perceptions. Likewise, if you believe poverty is your destiny and view wealth as out-of-reach or somehow repugnant, or if you believe that you are inherently unlucky, your beliefs will reinforce that experience.

Oddly, however, most people think things go in the opposite direction. They believe they are angry or disappointed in life because of random things that happened *to* them—job loss, divorce, etc. But what if Goddard is right and it actually goes the other way? What if our inner negativity and negative expectations literally create our negative outer experiences? Even if you superficially desire or intend something, if you are actually filled with doubt and self-loathing deep down inside, the world will reflect that deeper inner state of being. This may sound simplistic or too new-agey, but it's certainly something to consider.

That's why I said what I did at the beginning of this book; *in order to heal and achieve happiness and success, you must try to shift your inner state.* The rest of this book describes many tools and methods for achieving this kind of fundamental change. But the truth is, doing so can be difficult. Our negative states and expectations are usually ingrained habits that have been with us for a long time—usually since childhood. Because of this, our brains have literally been wired to reinforce them. So, it can take a lot of work to make a positive shift.

However, please note one thing. It's not about *forcing* a change, but rather, acknowledging where you're at, loving and accepting yourself as you are now, and then making a sincere attempt to grow. Indeed, as I've tried to stress, *that may be why we're here right now, incarnated into physical form at this time and place; to experience the things that will motivate us to make a shift.*

In other words, that's our purpose here on Earth. To experience, learn, and grow, and ideally, share our wisdom with others and help them too. In fact, we each literally selected our current incarnation with this purpose in mind—we signed up for it. This realization was a huge motivation and consolation to Steve and me when we decided to pick ourselves up, dismantle the life we had created in California for over 40 years, and find a new place, a new life. We recognized that everything over the course of the preceding 40 years had led us to take that step, and that ignoring this fact and staying in California out of habit, fear, and convenience was out of alignment with our life purpose.

Writer Mike Dooley[2] condenses the issue of life purpose into a simple formula. *Our purpose on Earth is to be happy.* This description may capture it all, because if you're negative, depressed, and angry, you won't be living a very happy life. Note too that Dooley doesn't mean the happiness of riches; everyone knows that the mega-wealthy are often miserable. As the old saw goes, "Money can't buy happiness." Moreover, studies have shown that one key path to happiness is through service—i.e., through *giving*, not receiving. In any case, if you *are* truly happy deep down inside, no matter what's going on in the outer world, you probably have found a way to transcend—that is, you've learned, likely over many lifetimes, *how* to be truly happy. Writer Anita Moorjani,[3] who survived a near-death experience from terminal cancer and then fully and miraculously healed, puts it another way: *Our purpose here on Earth is to love ourselves for who we are and shine our light brightly.*

What's the end game of all this? Perhaps, if we learn enough, we won't need to incarnate anymore. We might dwell for a while in the four-dimensional astral realm and become wise astral helpers for those living their astral life between physical lives. Eventually, we may even evolve to the point where we shed our Astral Body and become mental-causal beings living in the mental realm. Are we then angels, like the beings of light depicted in Nosso Lar? Is this a five-dimensional realm? Do we eventually become causal beings, united with the oneness of All That Is, or perhaps move on to even higher dimensional realms? Perhaps so.

Finally, is this strictly a one-way street? Do highly evolved beings ever decide to dwell among us here on three-dimensional planet Earth? Many people believe that they do—and that they incarnate on Earth in order to achieve some greater purpose—perhaps to guide and instruct humanity. These humans might be the people we know as Buddha, Moses, Jesus, or Lao Tsu.

The bottom line, of course, is that almost all of us have many incarnations ahead of us. We have a lot of learning left to do! So, let's move on to Part III and find out about some tools that will help you to do so in this lifetime.

PART III

FIND YOUR PATH TO HEALING

"The natural healing force within each one of us
is the greatest force in getting well."
–Hippocrates

CHAPTER 13

>–

HEALING
FROM THE OUTSIDE IN

Now that you understand the nature of the entire human being, comprised of the Physical Body, the energetic Etheric Body that sustains it, and the higher Astral, Mental, and Causal Bodies that accompany us from life to life, you can see why healing is definitely not just a physical affair.

In fact, more often than not, the true root of a health problem—even a very serious problem like cancer or heart disease—may not be within the Physical Body at all. As a result, modifying a body part through surgery or taking a pill to alter body chemistry may only serve as a palliative measure that alleviates but doesn't cure a problem. Of course, sometimes a physical intervention *is* necessary to save one's life. But all too often, what appears to cure a symptom may, in actuality, cause more dangerous symptoms down the line. This phenomenon, the negative result of symptom suppression, is well understood by most alternative medical practitioners, but it is generally lost on conventional doctors who view these negative results as "side effects" that need to be further medicated or simply endured.

MY OWN HEALING JOURNEY

What initially prompted me to write *Living in Synchrony* were some of my own experiences with illness. It all began with gastroesophageal reflux (GERD)—chronic heartburn that lasted for hours after each meal and felt like a nagging hunger pain in the pit of my stomach. Although these symptoms were alleviated by a change in diet, ultimately, I realized that my experience of GERD was rooted in deeper psychological issues—the same ones that led to my next and more challenging problem: chronic insomnia. As you will better understand after reading this book, my body had initially tried to tell me something that manifested as GERD. But because I had simply palliated the problem, I hadn't really listened to what it was trying to say. It then decided to afflict me with something I couldn't ignore as easily!

Anyone who has experienced chronic insomnia knows that the struggle for sleep can be as daunting and painful as many diseases. As weeks turned into months, my life became focused on how to make it through each day and face each night. In this weakened state, I didn't even have the energy to write a book. I also experienced chronic anxiety felt as tension in my abdomen, nights praying in the darkness for deliverance, and occasional suicidal feelings. Sometimes I resorted to sleeping pills—a painful step for someone like me who is committed to alternative medicine. In the darkness of night, I morbidly ruminated about celebrities who ultimately died from the same struggle for sleep—Michael Jackson, Heath Ledger, Marilyn Monroe, Judy Garland, and I'm sure many others.

My experience with severe insomnia lasted for over a year and continued as a more manageable issue for another year and a half. I still struggle at times, but it is mostly a thing of the past. During that period, I learned the wisdom of the old adage: *the only way out is through.* At first, I tried homeopathy (the subject of my first book), but it didn't help much. After a few months, I realized that I needed to embark upon an intense period of self-examination and soul-searching. I refused to accept that my insomnia was permanent or just an aspect of getting older. (By this point, I was in my 60s.) Instead, I sensed that it was a passageway into a new state of being.

The truth is, though, that the inner quest isn't easy for most people to engage in and most people won't. Perhaps they are afraid or are simply unable to penetrate within. But as a writer on alternative approaches to health and the evolution of consciousness, I simply had to try to do the work necessary to get to the other side. It felt wrong to follow in the footsteps of so many of my friends and become another cog in the medical machine, popping pills to get through another night. However, I also realized (eventually) that taking a pill occasionally, when I really needed it, was also a part of my growth. I had to learn to have more compassion for myself and let go of my chronic perfectionism and inner sense of guilt. More about that later.

Ever since I published my second book *Active Consciousness* in 2011, I have tried to follow my own intuitive guidance. For example, I have tried to choose my activities each day based on what sparks my interest, curiosity, and energy, and by what synchronicities or uncanny coincidences come my way. The first real spark that ultimately led to my writing the initial draft of *Living in Synchrony* was my discovery of Huna, the system of healing and spiritual practice I described earlier. I was browsing an alternative bookstore in Sebastopol, California when a thin little book on the subject suddenly grabbed my eye.[1] It was definitely a "ding! moment," as author Louise Hay used to say. After buying and reading it, I knew that Huna concepts were a part of my future. I particularly enjoyed the fact that they emphasized self-healing and echoed many of the ideas I wrote about in *Active Consciousness*. For a while, I thought *Living in Synchrony* would be a book about Huna, and I wrote several articles about the system. But my discovery of Huna was just the beginning.

At around the same time, I took a couple of workshops offered by the International Academy of Consciousness (IAC), which I also described earlier. My curiosity about the group had been piqued by a few friends who were avid participants in their programs. As discussed in Chapter 6, the IAC is based in Brazil and teaches techniques for achieving out-of-body experiences (OBEs). More fascinating to me, however, was the cosmology that the IAC teaches about what actually happens during an OBE. I found that their material rounded out information I was gleaning from Huna, and it also meshed well with the teachings of Rudolf Steiner and G.I. Gurdjieff, both of whom I wrote about in detail in *Active Consciousness*.

But Huna and the IAC were still only a beginning. In my quest to heal my insomnia, I explored many other healing modalities as well. They included hypnotherapy, the ideas and meditations found in Joe Dispenza's book *You are the Placebo*, the revolutionary Sedona Method, John Sarno's landmark work on the role of the subconscious in almost all forms of disease, and behavior modification therapy.

Another physical problem that developed for me during this same period, which no doubt was aggravated by chronic insomnia, was a tendency to have high blood pressure. Not wanting to start on medications for this condition (most of which have vast systemic side effects and are nearly impossible to discontinue), I started using a breathing technology called Resperate[2] that helps to lower blood pressure naturally. And when my tension during the COVID years aggravated my blood pressure further, especially after Steve and I realized that we needed to leave our California home of 38 years, I incorporated another stress reduction technique into my life—TRE (Trauma Release Exercises). I have found it to be transformational, and it also helps me to fall asleep! In addition, I learned a subtle word-based technique called Logosynthesis that I find quite helpful. Today, I still use TRE and Logosynthesis on a daily basis at bedtime.

Many other teachings and therapies have come into my life along the way. They include the work of teachers like Louise Hay and Kristin Neff on self-compassion, self-acceptance, and self-love. I have also read a lot of material on trust and manifestation, including the works of Florence Scovel Shinn, Neville Goddard, Tosha Silver, Ernest Holmes, Thomas Troward, and a book called *The Trust Frequency* by Andrew Cameron Bailey and Connie Baxter Marlow. Mike Dooley's book, *Life on Earth*, the well-known *A Course in Miracles*, and the writings of Anita Moorjani have also been helpful to me. Of course, these are merely the resources I have personally experienced; they are definitely not exhaustive. (See the Notes and Resources at the end of this book for more information and pointers.)

In summary, my advice is that when you experience any non-emergency form of physical, emotional or mental disease, pain, or other divergence from health, begin by pondering what the *true* root of your problem may actually be. Rather than rushing to a conventional medical doctor, who will feel obliged to "run tests" and prescribe some medication for you, your best first step might be to try a completely non-invasive and physically benign approach that addresses other parts of your complete being.

The rest of this chapter kicks off Part III by reviewing the various levels or layers at which problems can arise. Chapters 14—18 will then discuss each of these levels and its associated therapies in greater detail. Hopefully, this book will help you gain insight into how to address the true source of any particular dysfunction you may be experiencing.

THE LEVELS OF OUR BEING

Let's begin by looking at the table below. Following the model I discussed in Chapter 11, I've organized the levels of our complete being from the physical realm inward. The physical level includes all of the tissues, organ systems, and fluids of the Physical Body—the biological machine of our existence. We then move inward to the Etheric Body, the energy framework upon which the Physical Body is built. Finally, we consider the higher Astral, Mental, and Causal Bodies that continue on after we die.

	BODY	**MILIEU**
PHYSICAL	Organs and physical tissues and fluids, physical injuries, habitual or repetitive behaviors, posture, sleep	Diet, physical environment (including other people, animals, plants, toxins, moisture, light, heat, cold, mold, dryness), living and work conditions, drugs, vaccines, bacteria and viruses and other microbiota (both inside and outside the body)
ETHERIC	Qi or vital force, chakras, meridians	Etheric Bodies of the physical milieu (including those of other people, plants, animals, and microbiota), electromagnetic fields
ASTRAL	Emotions, memories, psychic perceptions, past-life memories, emotional habits	Astral Bodies of other people and animals, and possibly plants and other aspects of the environment, nature spirits, other astral beings

MENTAL	Thoughts, rational thinking abilities, will, imagination, creativity, meaning	Mental Bodies of other people and possibly animals, plants, and other aspects of the environment, other mental beings
CAUSAL	Spirit, wisdom, love, serenity, connection to inner knowing, ability to manifest and create	Causal Bodies of other people and other causal beings

The Levels of Our Complete Being

Notice that the levels in the table include not only what we consider to be "us," but also what we consider to be "not us"—that is, the environment in which we live at a particular level. For example, our Physical Body is embedded within a physical environment. Each environment is essentially a "stew" in which we are inextricably interconnected with everything else. For this reason, I will tend to use the term "milieu" instead of "environment" for the rest of this book. The word "milieu" has been likened to the word "atmosphere" and can also be used to denote a cultural setting, not just a physical one. It thus seems more appropriate than "environment," which has a more exterior and physical connotation. As we will see, *all* levels of our being are embedded in a milieu, whether it be physical, etheric, astral, mental, or causal. That's why addressing the milieu of a particular level may be just as important as addressing what is specifically "us." In other words, we need to get in synchrony not only within, but also without—at all levels. Chapter 19 considers all of the milieus in more detail.

EACH LEVEL HAS INHERENT HEALING POWER

As we go from the physical realm inward toward the causal level of our being, the inherent healing power of each level increases. For instance, healing your Etheric Body has more power to create overall health than merely addressing your Physical Body alone. Similarly, healing at the astral level has more inherent power than healing at the physical or etheric levels. And the power of the mental level is truly awesome! We all know that the sheer will to heal and to live can enable someone to do so against all odds. Finally, there is the all-powerful ability of the causal level to create healing miracles.

Much more evidence for what I am saying will be covered in the chapters that follow. Each will focus on a particular level and will include:

- Indicators that a particular problem exists at that level.

- Indicators that the root of a problem does *not* exist at that level and suggestions for where it might be rooted.

- Pointers to various therapies and techniques that operate on that level.

- Cautions to keep in mind when using therapies addressing that level.

Of course, many times, a problem exists at multiple levels. Similarly, many therapies address multiple levels at once. Why? Because all of our physical and energy bodies are interconnected. That's why astral or mental healing can penetrate into your Etheric Body and through it, affect your Physical Body too. That's why physical healing methods can affect your Etheric Body and thereby the emotions and mind of your Astral and Mental Bodies. And that's why etheric healing modalities like homeopathy or acupuncture are so powerful—because they easily reach into the Physical and the Higher Energy Bodies.

What has determined my categorization of treatments in this book? Mostly, it is the underlying philosophy of the system, how it is typically utilized in practice, what tools it uses, and the kinds of ailments it is usually used to address. For instance, chiropractors see their treatment as primarily correcting physical problems in the spine, even if they also recognize the existence of the Etheric Body. Nevertheless, the categories I have chosen aren't locked in stone.

It is also important to realize that a healing technique that focuses on one level can be limited or stymied by dysfunction at another level. For example, if your leg is deeply gashed or broken, there is only so much that changing your beliefs (Astral Body) will accomplish. You still need to stitch up the skin and set the bone. Or, even if you have a very strong *will* to heal (Mental Body) but deep down inside you don't *believe* you can (Astral Body)—possibly because a doctor has given you strong a "nocebo" or negative message and has told you that healing is impossible—you will likely not be able to do so.

That's why you need to try to live in synchrony overall and address issues and blockages at all levels for true healing success. For example, if you want to be truly successful at manifesting at the causal level (for example, by using the Ha Ritual described in Chapter 9), you first need to address unconscious aspects of your Astral Body that may be blocking you. And even if you are working on releasing unconscious beliefs and are going to an acupuncturist or homeopath to work on your Etheric Body, it is still important to clean up your diet and get some exercise!

So, let's begin with the first and most obvious place to get things in order: your Physical Body and its physical milieu.

CHAPTER 14

WE ARE PHYSICAL BEINGS

Each of us has decided to incarnate into a Physical Body. We might deny the demands of our physical vessel in myriad ways, but in the end, it will make itself heard. Our needs as little babies remain with us throughout life. We feel hunger and thirst and heat and cold and dryness and moisture. We must urinate and defecate. We need sleep. We get sick. And ultimately, our Physical Body dies.

Nevertheless, most of us often neglect our bodily needs; we get out of sync with our physical being. We indulge all too often in fast foods and sugary treats. We refuse to make time for exercise and eventually lose strength and agility as a result. We develop a variety of addictions that place a huge strain on our Physical Bodies. We ignore important bodily alarm signals when we become overly absorbed in work, sporting successes, or even a spiritual quest.

So how can we heal the body? While it is true that non-physically-based methods can work miracles on the physical level, it is also true that there are limits to what can be achieved if we completely neglect our physical frame. On the other hand, most people seem to think that physical means of healing are the *only* means. Or they confine themselves to only one or two methods—conventional modern medicine being the primary choice. Luckily, many people are reexamining this approach, as its limitations and costs increasingly become felt.

For so many reasons, then, it is important to consider a broad array of healing options and to learn about the upsides and downsides of each, along with its suitability in various circumstances. The physically-based methods I will cover in this chapter include not only conventional medicine, but also many alternative or complementary therapies that treat the body in a physical, non-energetic way. They include nutrition, detoxification, herbalism, and strategies that physically manipulate the body. The possibilities are vast, so I will only touch upon the ones I am personally familiar with. This will also be true of the chapters that focus on the nonphysical realms. My goal is to be illustrative, not exhaustive. Finally, in addition to describing many therapies, I will cover three other things to keep in mind:

1. Signs that a problem is likely rooted in the physical realm.

2. Signs that a problem is likely *not* rooted in this realm (along with ideas about where the root might be).

3. Cautions to keep in mind while pursuing any particular technique.

So let's begin!

SIGNS AND CAUTIONS FOR THE PHYSICAL REALM

Your body feels unwell, you are anxious or depressed, or you are experiencing pain. Where to turn? What approach should you take? Before you run off to a medical doctor, alternative practitioner, or decide to ignore it, here are some things to keep in mind.

Signs that your problem may be physically based:

- The problem began with an injury to the body or some kind of organ damage.

- You were exposed to bad food, toxins, mold, a difficult weather situation, drugs, a contagious disease, or something new or unusual in the outer world.

- The problem responds well to physically-based treatment, and you continue to feel better without ongoing treatment. In other words, if a healer tells you that you need to keep coming back indefinitely or take a pill forever, you should also begin to look deeper for answers.

Signs that the problem is not purely physical and might be helped by nonphysical approaches:

- The problem is transient and keeps moving around to different parts of the body.

- Physical treatment is palliative or suppressive—it doesn't hold and must be repeated indefinitely.

- The severity of the problem is out of proportion to the supposed injury or is ascribed to something that was never a problem before.

- The problem began after an emotional upset or some other psychologically traumatic event.

Cautions:

- Try less invasive tests and treatments first.

- Try one treatment at a time (ideally, for at least a couple of weeks) to see if it really helps. Avoid panic and using a "shotgun" approach (trying many things at once), which can lead to confusion and possibly indecipherable side effects and interactions.

- Make sure that any tests you undergo are useful, safe, and can actually lead to treatment possibilities, not just more "information" for a practitioner. Unfortunately, many unnecessary and invasive tests have become standard procedure in conventional medicine. Sometimes they are done only to avoid liability claims or to follow organizational directives that may not be in the best interest of individual patients. So do your homework and ask questions.

- Be aware and wary of side effects. These have become pervasive in conventional medicine due to the overuse of medications, drug interactions, and treatments that are suppressive, not curative. Once again, do your homework and exercise caution.

- Avoid suppression when possible, especially if doing so is merely for your own convenience. Try to give your body the opportunity to heal on its own.

- Think deeply about recent exposures to noxious influences (both physical and emotional). These exposures are clues that may lead you to the true root of your problem, and they are often ignored or glossed over by many doctors.

- Don't be influenced by "nocebos"—negative or hopeless messages or pronouncements from doctors or therapists, especially if you are generally healthy. *Remember that such messages deeply affect your Astral*

Body and can actually keep you from healing! Instead, believe in your body's ability to heal.

PHYSICALLY-BASED THERAPIES

Physically-based healing tools are the ones most people are familiar with and that we tend to utilize most often. These tools are also the most well-developed and widespread—and that's only natural. We live in a physical world and when a problem arises, the most obvious solution is to address it physically.

Below is a list of approaches I'll cover in this chapter. I've grouped them into two categories—ones that *add or subtract* something to the body, and those that operate via *external movement or manipulation.* Please note that some practitioners (especially alternative practitioners like chiropractors, osteopaths, and naturopaths) often utilize techniques that address the nonphysical levels too, especially the Etheric Body (the subject of Chapter 15). This is also true of yoga and some massage techniques.

Approaches that add something to or subtract something from your body:

- Conventional medicine (surgery and drugs)

- Diet and supplementation

- Herbalism

- Detoxification

Approaches that externally move or manipulate your body and its organs:

- Exercise

- Physical therapy

- Posture therapies

- Movement therapies

- Massage

- Chiropractic

- Osteopathy, Craniosacral therapy

Approaches that add something to or subtract something from your body

Conventional Medicine (surgery and drugs)

There's no doubt that conventional "modern" medicine (also known as *allopathy*) is now the dominant healing approach used in the world today. With all of its high tech gadgetry, surgical prowess, and an unending stream of pharmaceutical drugs, it's where most of us tend to run first, especially in an emergency. And it is precisely in emergency situations—treating wounds, performing surgeries—that allopathy truly excels. If you are hit by a car or break your leg, by all means, run to the doctor or hospital. In these circumstances, the wonders of modern medicine are lifesavers.

The supreme dominance of what we now call "conventional" medicine developed in the 1900s, with the rise of the pharmaceutical industry and the availability of fairly reliable drugs—especially painkillers, antibiotics, and vaccines. Before that, doctors had limited success, especially in epidemics. That is why a variety of other approaches were used and often were more successful and prominent. One prime example is my own favorite, *homeopathy*—an inherently etheric form of medicine that will be discussed in Chapter 15. Other more physically-based modalities that were popular in the 1800s include herbalism, chiropractic, and osteopathy. All of them worked when conventional medicine was helpless, and they still work well today.

As the power of the pharmaceutical industry grew, however, alternative healing methods were shut out and often banned. For example, while there were homeopathic medical crews tending to soldiers in World War I, by World War II, the American homeopathic medical schools had been shuttered or converted into allopathic schools. Eventually, the public's belief that a conventional doctor could provide "a pill for every ill" grew to be almost complete.

As is often the case with human beings, we tend to go too far and get too cocky in our hubris. Thus, it is only recently that people have come to realize that the overuse of antibiotics and other drugs comes at a price and may, in fact, be destroying our health. For example, it is only in the past 10-20 years that scientists have begun to realize how important good bacteria, viruses, and fungi are in determining our health. These *microbiota* dwell not only in the environment and within our guts, but can also be found throughout our bodies. In fact, they may be what's usually running the show—perhaps even more so than our genes. The critters that live within us must be fed and nourished by nontoxic foods, which our human bodies evolved to require—not eradicated by the overuse of antivirals, antibiotics, and fungicides.

Unfortunately, this wisdom has been lost in our rush to modernity and convenience. In essence, we got out of sync with our bodies and our environment. Sadly, most conventional doctors are still unaware of the latest research on microbiota. They also tend to have limited training in nutrition and are often unwary of the danger in killing off their patients' microbiomes with antibiotics and other drugs. And let's not forget that antibiotic agents are endemic in household products and are widely used in food production too, especially in meat production. The result has been havoc in our bodies and the advent of antibiotic resistance—a leading cause of deaths from hospital infections. Gone are the days when hospitals were the safest and most sterile environments. Now, undergoing surgery comes with a growing risk of infection.

Of course, conventional doctors aren't malicious; they have simply been trained in a system that, over the years, has become increasingly specialized, erratic, and influenced by the companies that make the latest gadgets and pills. Indeed, the standards of practice and the array of available drugs are constantly changing. Simultaneously, it has been shown that medical school training tends to lag significantly behind the latest research. In contrast, traditional "alternative" therapies tend to be quite stable. Thus, the tools of homeopathy, herbalism, chiropractic, and traditional osteopathy have remained largely the same as they were one hundred years ago. They worked then and they still work now.

One key reason for the current failures and outrageous costs of modern medicine (especially in the treatment of chronic disease) is that it depends on drugs that largely suppress the symptoms of disease rather than cure them. A typical example is the use of steroid creams for eczema. Although such creams can succeed in making eczema disappear, it often returns, and if not, can lead to deeper systemic problems like allergies. If allergies are then also suppressed, they can lead to asthma. Doctors know that such progressions are common, but they do not recognize that the underlying cause may be suppressive treatment; in contrast, many alternative practitioners do.

Never-ending pill-popping may be lucrative for drug companies, but it isn't helpful to patients and their pocketbooks. The drug companies churn out more products each year, and it has been estimated that a third of these products will be deemed harmful and pulled from the market later on.[1] Nevertheless, because we are constantly bombarded by pharmaceutical advertisements that tout the latest "medical miracle," we are tempted to resort to pill-popping without thinking about the possible side-effects—despite the fact that these effects are murmured quickly and quietly at the end of each advertisement, just in case you decide to file a lawsuit.

As a result, so many of us manage our anxiety or depression with drugs rather than trying to figure out a deeper reason (or a more benign solution) for our woes. We use pills to treat acne or to lower cholesterol rather than changing our diet. And rather than trying to meditate or diet naturally, we take even more pills to lower our blood pressure and to lose weight. Sadly, it is typical for the medical industry to foster this pattern. For example, medical authorities (funded by the pharmaceutical companies) have steadily lowered the bar of what "normal" blood pressure is each year, rendering most adults candidates for more pills.

Today, most of us have simply forgotten the teachings of older and more traditional methods of healing that always recognized that unending suppression leads to deeper, more chronic disease. As a result, the majority of adults and even children are now chronically ill and are taking way too many medications, which in turn make them even sicker. In fact, that may be the very reason you are reading this book—to learn another way.

Luckily, there *are* other ways, even within the physical realm, and most of them do not act suppressively. Rather than trying to force the body to alter its chemistry, these approaches generally try to support the *inherent healing ability of the Physical Body itself.* In other words, they operate in synchrony *with* the body, not against it. After all, human beings (and all living beings) are naturally self-healing. We wouldn't be here if that weren't true. Millennia of human beings have survived on Earth without the benefit of modern drugs! The next time you cut your finger, be sure to wash it and bandage it, and then observe and marvel at that way it heals over the next few days. Your body and its assistants, the microbiota, are truly miraculous.

In truth, most of the time, your "symptoms" are just signs that your body is making an effort to heal you. That's *why* you develop a fever—to kill off and eliminate harmful bacteria. That's *why* you get a blister when you burn—to protect and provide nutrients to the burned area as it heals. The body is always making an effort to heal itself. Of course, that doesn't mean it can't use a little help sometimes. When you need a conventional doctor to save your life, please do call upon them. But if a more benign approach or just plain bed rest is sufficient, try that first. There are also scores of other therapies within the physical realm that can come to your aid. Let's consider some of them.

Diet and Supplementation

The most natural and obvious approach to improving physical health is with food. As the adage goes, "You are what you eat." Or as computer scientists say, "Garbage in, garbage out." The paramount importance of diet has been a mainstay of healing for millennia. Sadly, most doctors receive just a few hours of instruction about nutrition in medical school, and hospitals are notorious for serving unwholesome food, even as patients are desperately trying to heal.

Actually, changing your diet is probably the safest and often the most powerful approach to any health problem and therefore the most logical thing to try first. As Hippocrates said, "Let food be thy medicine." Maimonides (a famed Jewish philosopher and doctor from the 12th century who lived in Spain and Egypt) agreed. He advised, "No disease that can be treated by diet should be treated with any other means." Maimonides also stressed the importance of not overeating. Here are some more quotes from him that we should all take to heart today:

- "One should not eat until his stomach is full. Rather, [he should stop eating when] he has eaten close to three quarters of his full satisfaction."

- "Overeating is like poison to anyone's body. It is the main source of all illness. Most illnesses which afflict a man are caused by harmful foods or by his filling his stomach and overeating, even of healthful foods."

- "Do not eat unless you're hungry."

Wise words!

Of course, many people are becoming aware of the need to eat more healthfully. One reason is that a growing number of people have become sensitized to and sickened by foods that were once considered dietary mainstays: wheat, dairy, peanuts, and more. Allergies are skyrocketing. EpiPens now adorn the walls of summer camps. When I attended a summer camp in Canada in the 1960s, the infirmary consisted of a few rooms on the second floor of a small building. Today, that same camp has constructed a veritable medical complex, housed in what was once the largest meeting hall. A huge number of campers now line up each day for their meds.

Why has this happened? There are many reasons. First and foremost may be the growing toxicity of our food supply. In many ways, what happened to conventional medicine during the 1900s was mirrored and magnified within the agricultural industry during that same time period. Because of the increasing power and short-term successes of the pharmaceutical industry, humanity began to believe that plants and soil could and should be engineered in the same way—by using plant drugs if you will. As a result, agricultural practices became dominated by the use of artificial fertilizers and pesticides—many of which were waste byproducts of weapons development and in some cases, were even used as biological weapons.

Unfortunately, dumping these wastes onto our farmlands also became a convenient and lucrative way of disposing of them. Along the same lines, the addition of fluoride to our water supplies has been touted as a way of preventing tooth decay. But if you investigate this practice more fully, you will discover that fluoride is an industrial waste product that is *not* healthy for your body, your brain, or your teeth. Luckily, decades of pushback by informed consumers is starting to have an effect.

In any case, over the course of the 1900s, farmers became convinced (and in some cases, coerced) to ignore the natural agricultural methods that had been developed for thousands of years. Temporary gains in crop yield (analogous to quick fixes via medical drugs) eventually led to dangerous soil depletion worldwide, the growth of superweeds, and a food supply that is poisoning us (analogous to the increasing incidence of chronic disease in humans, caused by suppression and the overuse of antibiotics).

Actually, these aren't just analogies. It turns out that plants survive and operate much the same way animals do. It is only recently that plant biologists are beginning to understand this. Naturally, farmers have been trying to understand how plants grow since the advent of agriculture. But it is only since the turn of the new millennium that we are discovering that, just as in our own bodies, *it is the invisible microbiota living in the soil that are really running the show.*

For many years, a plant's roots were believed to be the only things that enabled them to take up minerals and other nutrients from soil. We are now discovering, however, that the roots exude sugars, which then attract microbiota to them. These invisible microscopic workers—which make up half of all life on the planet and have been around a lot longer than any plant or animal—then break down soil constituents and deliver nutrients to the roots. But when we apply toxic pesticides to the soil, the microbiota are killed! The result: toxified food that is increasingly devoid of the nutrition we require.

A parallel mechanism is going on within us. Just as in the soil, the microbiota in our guts—our *microbiome*—break down the foods we eat, thereby making nutrients available to us. But when we poison or kill this internal factory by ingesting poisoned foods, toxic drugs, or antibiotics, this process is hampered. The lining of our guts becomes weakened and more permeable, allowing indigestible food particles to enter our bloodstream. The net effect? We become sensitized or allergic to the foods we eat the most: wheat and dairy. After all, the body is merely trying to defend itself from indigestible particles. But without sufficient nutrition, the body's defenses slowly break down too and chronic diseases develop. When we simultaneously expose our already weakened bodies to other environmental toxins, we inevitably increase the havoc.

So, it's definitely time to try to heal our microbiome! Luckily, diet and supplementation are key ways to do so. Don't forget, our bodies are resilient self-healing wonders. The soil is too. With knowledge and effort, we can eliminate toxins and rebuild soils and our bodies. Techniques for healing the human microbiome are still in their infancy, but many now believe that a variety of fairly benign modalities may be effective solutions. Indeed, it's imperative that we *do* solve this problem, because a disturbed microbiome can contribute to many chronic diseases that are becoming increasingly common: obesity, diabetes, heart disease, cancer, food sensitivities, neurological diseases like MS, ALS, Parkinson's, Alzheimers, ADD/ADHD, and autism, as well as depression and anxiety.

Right now, there aren't that many practitioners who specialize in addressing the microbiome. So if this seems like an approach you'd like to try, your best bet is to see a functional or integrative doctor or a naturopath. Some conventionally trained nutritionists might also be up on the latest research. But at this point, most of these practitioners will simply provide you with some general tips: try a gluten-free or dairy-free diet, eliminate common problem foods and allergens, and take supplements. Unfortunately, these may just be band-aid solutions because they only try to eliminate the foods that aggravate you (letting your gut rest and heal) and add in vitamins, minerals, and other nutrients to make up the difference.

A more complete approach is to actively heal the gut itself and restore a healthy microbiome. Towards that end, some doctors are experimenting with fecal transplants, implanting a small amount of the microbiome of a healthy person into the gut of a sick person. This has had remarkable results in cases of Crohn's disease and colitis. In general, though, the best first approach is to change your diet and feed the good microbiota within your microbiome by consuming *prebiotics*. These are foods that your microbiome loves. The most important prebiotic foods are fermented items like sauerkraut, kimchi, and yogurt. That's why so many traditional diets include them.

It is also critical to realize that stress—your emotions and even your thoughts—directly affects your microbiome. You literally *are* what you think and feel. Your thoughts and feelings affect your microbiome, and your microbiome runs your body. And it goes the other way too! Your gut microbiota affect and create brain chemicals that influence your thoughts and feelings. Do you think that you need to take an antidepressant? You might be better off changing your diet. Eat some sauerkraut before each meal instead!

Once your gut is fed and flowing a bit more normally, it can also be helpful to take *probiotics*, supplements that contain good microbiota. Just a few years ago, practitioners believed that probiotics re-supplied the microbiome, much like adding fuel to a tank. However, it is now emerging that the microbiome is much more complex than we realized, with thousands of different microbiota performing functions we barely understand. Some scientists now believe that probiotics simply add new agents into this mix, thereby minimizing the influence of bad biota and increasing the power of the good. But *how* probiotics truly affect the microbiome is still food for future research (pun intended!).

Because of the inherent complexity of the human microbiome, studying its individual components may be nearly an impossible task. One recent approach, however, is to utilize the statistical power of artificial intelligence. A company called Viome is now collecting fecal samples from those who sign up for its services. They then analyze the DNA and RNA of the microbiomes in these samples and try to derive statistical conclusions about the makeup of healthy versus unhealthy microbiomes. The company is also trying to correlate certain microbiome patterns with specific diseases.[2] Based on these results, Viome customers are given advice about particular prebiotic foods to eat and probiotic supplements to take. This kind of work is still in its infancy, but it's a start. At the same time, I am personally wary of the invasion of privacy and bodily autonomy that such AI-based efforts exemplify. So, proceed with caution.

If you're keen to start working on your diet on your own, there are scores of diets you can try. Truthfully, I'm not an expert on any of them. Some may be good for some people, some may not be. My recommendation is to explore online, try things out, and see what feels right for you and your body. Remember: not all bodies and not all microbiomes are alike! Indeed, one ancient system of medicine that recognizes human variability in dietary needs is Ayurveda, a traditional medicine from India. Many of you have probably heard of it because of the popularity of Deepak Chopra's first book, *Perfect Health*, which focuses on Ayurveda.[3] In fact, it was that book that first got me interested in alternative forms of medicine.

Ayurveda recognizes three main types of constitution—Vata, Pitta, and Kapha—with most people falling into a mixture of these categories. Determining one's type is a holistic process, based on physical and emotional characteristics. Depending on your constitutional type, different diets, herbs, and practices like massage are then recommended. For instance, some people are advised to eat cold and raw foods, while others benefit from warm and sweet foods. You might think of this approach as a way of aligning or syncing your diet with your overall nature.

Exotic diets and practices aside, perhaps the easiest first thing to try is to improve your diet with the following simple guidelines. They can help anyone live in synchrony with their innate requirements as a physical being:

- **Drink water.** Many of the disease symptoms people experience today are simply the result of dehydration. In fact, dehydration is especially common in the elderly and is the root of many of their problems. Remove sodas from your diet and replace them with water, or if you must have a soda sometimes, try carbonated water with a bit of juice. Not only is excess sugar toxic to your system, but it also feeds cancer and other diseases. Be aware that sugar replacements (and diet sodas) are even worse than sugar because they poison your microbiome. In fact, many sugar replacements were originally developed as pesticides.

- **Avoid all genetically-modified (GMO) foods and eat organic whenever possible.** Most GMO foods have been engineered to be resistant to pesticides and thus are literally bathed in them. Some GMO foods are even designed to manufacture their own pesticides internally! When you eat these foods, you are literally eating pesticides and killing your microbiome in the process. One of the most toxic and pervasive pesticides is *glyphosate* (Roundup), which is now found in the umbilical cords of newborn babies. The growing use of glyphosate has also been statistically correlated with the growth rate of many chronic diseases that we are experiencing today, including autism.

- **Prepare your own food.** Not only will you eat more nutritiously and know what you're actually eating, but the aromas you experience while cooking activate your digestive enzymes, which prepare your microbiome for efficient digestion. You may also find that eating what you cook at home is the easiest way to lose weight.

- **Food is ultimately a better source of nutrition than supplements.** Indeed, supplements should be used sparingly and only when your diet falls short in some way. For one thing, you know what's in your food; it's harder to know what's in your supplements. In addition, most supplements only provide some of a food's constituents, whereas a whole food is composed of many elements that can have important synergistic effects. Of course, supplementation is sometimes necessary. But food can often suffice and is preferable in most cases.

- **Go outside.** Take a walk in nature. Expose yourself to dirt and your skin to sunlight (the best source of vitamin D)—ideally without the use of toxic sunscreens. Grow your own vegetables, pick them up off the ground, and eat them. By simply exposing yourself to fresh air and the great outdoors, you will not only feel better emotionally, but you also help to seed your microbiome with healthy microbiota.

- **Eat lots of prebiotic foods that help to feed a healthy microbiome.** For example, try to eat more fiber, whole vegetables and fruits, root vegetables, beans, legumes, resistant starch, fermented foods, and good fats like avocado. Avoid refined sugar and flour, all ultra-processed foods, factory-farm raised meats (full of antibiotics), and excessive alcohol. Note: drinking more than two alcoholic drinks per day is definitely harmful to your microbiome; less is even better.

- **Alleviate stress using the many healing strategies described throughout this book—especially meditation.** Remember that your emotional state and even your thoughts directly affect your microbiome.

Herbal Medicine

Most of us have heard of herbalism—the medicinal practice of ingesting or applying tinctures, teas, poultices, etc. derived from plant material. It is the oldest form of healing on Earth. Even animals know which plants to eat when they have an upset stomach. Our Physical Bodies are animals too and evolved to live successfully on this planet. Since plants were here long before we were, we naturally evolved so that we could survive and heal by utilizing them.

For example, the plant foods that grow in specific areas and times of year tend to be the ones most perfect for our needs. Think of citrus fruits, which provide a wonderful supply of vitamin C during the cold season. Or berries, which do the same for us during the summer. Today's microbiome scientists believe that locally grown foods are even better for us, because they best suit our microbiome. Thus, someone living in the Pacific Northwest will benefit more from foods that grow naturally there than from foods that have been grown in the tropics.

Even more amazing is that the plants that tend to grow in certain areas are often perfect for the kinds of injuries that can occur there. *Arnica Montana* springs to mind—a little yellow mountain flower that is used herbally as well as in ultradilute homeopathic preparations as a premier solution for bumps and bruises. It's just the thing you might need when you are trekking along a stony mountain path and suffer a fall. Did Arnica Montana spring up beneficently just to aid us? Or did we co-evolve with it? Our inherent interrelationships with plants are certainly an example of how we are healed when we live in synchrony with our environment.

Every culture on Earth has developed some form of herbalism to cure its ailments. There are Chinese herbalists, Native American herbalists, the herbal healers of the Amazon, and those throughout Europe (especially before allopathic medicine took over). Today, herbalism is an important part of holistic medical systems that are practiced by doctors all over the world—for example, Chinese medicine and India's Ayurveda. And just as is still true today, many of the herbal healers of the past were women—healers who were once branded as "witches." Shamans are also herbal healers and utilize techniques that address the Etheric and Higher Energy Bodies too.

Although herbalism is considered to be "alternative" by today's allopathic doctors, it is actually the *original* physically-based form of medicine. Grounded in wisdom and experience that has been developed and tested for thousands of years, it has healed humanity for millennia. None of us would be here without it! Although new plants may be discovered, the treatments used by herbalists thousands of years ago are still valid today. And although the chemicals found in them may sometimes act by suppressing symptoms, in general they operate by stimulating the body's natural healing abilities.

In fact, many of the ingredients in today's pharmaceuticals are based upon plants used by herbalists. Unfortunately, in the pharmaceutical industry's materialistic rush to utilize and monopolize this knowledge, it did not recognize that plants are not simply bags of chemicals. They are living beings that carry a variety of synergistic elements and energies within them that contribute to their healing power. In other words, plants act not only physically, but at higher energy levels too. Herbalists understand this and so do homeopaths, who capture this energy using their unique remedy preparation methodology. But when pharmaceutical companies replace plant ingredients with artificially-derived chemical equivalents, or use them in strengths that humans did not evolve to tolerate, problems can arise.

If you feel like you would like to try herbalism as a solution to a health problem, please remember that herbal preparations can be powerful agents, just as pharmaceutical drugs are. They are not harmless simply because they are "natural." Moreover, each person's susceptibility and response to herbal products can be different. For this reason, it is always wise to utilize this form of medicine under the guidance of a trained and certified herbalist.

One type of practitioner that is trained in herbalism is a *naturopath*. Naturopaths were once called "eclectic" doctors because they use a variety of healing techniques, including herbal medicine. Some of today's naturopaths (called naturopathic physicians) have gained licensure and their services might be covered by health insurance. Other types of practitioners who utilize herbalism include functional or integrative medical doctors, chiropractors, acupuncturists, Ayurvedic doctors, and traditional Chinese doctors. Another option is to seek out someone who specializes strictly in herbalism. Ask around, use the internet. Always use your intuition and judgment when choosing a practitioner, as well as in deciding how long you should continue using this or any other form of treatment.

Detoxification

So far, I have talked about physically-based healing methods that focus on *adding* something into or onto the Physical Body, whether it be pharmaceuticals, foods, or herbal preparations. But there are also times when a problem is caused by toxins—for example, pesticides like glyphosate or mercury that is present in our air, food, and other products. Or, perhaps you drank polluted water or came into contact with toxic soil or black mold. You might also become sick because of lead in paint or poisons present in foods or drugs that have been ingested or injected. You might even have been bitten by a venomous insect or snake. Whatever the cause, sometimes it's simply necessary to remove the offending substance. That's what detoxification is all about.

The first step to take when you suspect something is toxic is to get away from it. Stop eating foods that you are allergic to. Stop using detergents, makeup, or other products that cause reactions. Stop drinking polluted water and clean up the mold in your house. Avoid (as best you can) fluoridated water and toothpaste and foods with pesticides, preservatives, and dyes.

Nevertheless, remember that, while exposure to external toxins is not great, *you are a powerful healing entity*. Humanity has always suffered from toxic exposures; it's not just a modern problem. In order to survive, your Physical Body possesses mechanisms that help it to resist, filter out, expel, and heal from noxious influences. Many of your organs and your overall immune system are specifically designed for this task. In essence, you were designed to regain a positive vibration, even when you are bombarded by an unsettling one. So, the techniques listed below for detoxification simply enhance the power your body already possesses to detoxify.

Also, don't forget that help can be found by using therapies that work on the etheric and higher levels too. Just because an external toxin is physical doesn't mean that you need to use a physically-based method to deal with it. For example, your mind and emotions have a powerful influence upon your immune functions, your microbiome, and your organ functionality, and thus, on your ability to detox. You'll learn more about such techniques in the ensuing chapters.

My personal favorite of these energy-based detoxification tools is *homeopathy*, an etheric form of medicine that has a long and successful track record in stimulating physical detoxification. One common approach that homeopaths use is to give a remedy made from the toxic offender itself. A unique technique called *potentization* captures the energetic signature of a toxin, which is then given to the patient. There are several illustrations of this method in my book *Impossible Cure*. One is the story of a dental hygienist who successfully expelled mercury in her menstrual blood by taking a remedy made from mercury. Another recounts the experience of an apple orchardist on the verge of death from arsenic poisoning. Thanks to homeopathic treatment, he sweated out huge amounts of the substance in a short period of time. Somehow, an energetic dose of these substances stimulates the Physical Body to expel them.

Naturally, there are dozens of physically-based methods of detoxification too. Although I am not an expert in any of them, I have provided a short list of methods to explore below. Aside from getting good sleep, drinking lots of water, eating healthy foods, and exercising, it is probably wise to enlist a trained expert if you think you need help with detoxification. Naturopaths are a good place to start.

Common detoxification strategies include the following:

- Sleep is your body's most important method of detoxification— healing body, emotions, and mind.

- Drink lots of water to flush out toxins via your kidneys, and eat foods that help cleanse your colon.

- Exercise and other forms of movement help to promote blood flow and detoxification through sweating.

- Water-based therapies, such as soaking in mineral baths, sitting in saunas or steam rooms, and sweat lodges can all be helpful. Most eliminate toxins via sweating. There are also many water-based techniques that can be useful in healing colds and flus.

- Superheating or supercooling the body can promote specific internal detoxification functions.

- The use of plant or mineral-based poultices applied to the skin can draw out toxins. This approach is particularly useful when dealing with infections and animal poisons. I once used both plant and mineral-based poultices to help heal a troublesome centipede bite.

- A variety of antioxidants and supplements (including some that are used intravenously) can be used to detoxify.

- Fasting can trigger detox. For example, juice fasts have been used to heal a variety of chronic ailments created by our unhealthy modern diets. Supervised water fasts have been reported to "reboot" the entire system and heal patients with serious diseases like cancer and diabetes.

- Many people cleanse their organs, including the liver, kidney, and gall bladder, by taking oral preparations made from herbs and oils. Also in this category is colonic irrigation.

- The use of oxygen and other gases via hyperbaric oxygen chambers, ozone therapy, and hydrogen-infused water (a potent antioxidant) can all help the body to detoxify.

- The internal use of minerals like activated charcoal and zeolite can bind to toxins so that they can then be excreted. Chelation is an aggressive form of this kind of therapy and should only be pursued under professional guidance.

Approaches that externally manipulate your body and its organs and systems

So far, I have discussed a variety of methods that utilize some external agent, be it a drug, food, or skin application. Sometimes, however, simply moving your physical frame around can do the trick. So many of us think we need to find someone who can fix our problems with a "magic bullet." When we think this way, we are forgetting two things: 1) Our very physical form—the shape and movements of our Physical Body—deeply affects what's going on inside it; and 2) We can be our own most powerful healer. For example, poor posture can impede your breathing, which then limits your oxygen intake and, as a consequence, the functionality of your entire body. That's why you can often get the most "bang for your buck" by simply changing your physical habits. This kind of approach may not be quick and expedient, but it certainly can be the deepest, safest, and most life changing.

Many of the completely benign and non-invasive approaches that I'll describe below have helped me tremendously. They saved me from surgery, healed troublesome tingling on the right side of my body, and alleviated neck, back, and jaw pain. Some have become quite popular, but others are less well-known. I urge you to find out if any of them might be helpful to you.

Exercise and Physical Therapy

This category of treatment needs little explanation. I'm sure you already realize that your Physical Body is held up, protected, and controlled by your bones, muscles, ligaments, and tendons. If you let your muscles atrophy, you will simply not be able to move around very well anymore. And if you cannot move, your blood flow will be poor and *all* of your organs, including your brain, will suffer.

Also remember that strong muscles can compensate for many physical weaknesses—for example, torn or stretched out ligaments. Anyone who has an elderly family member knows that falls can precipitate serious health problems. We may make jokes about the emergency "buttons" that the elderly use to tell someone, "I've fallen and can't get up!", but why can't they get up? It's because their muscles have become too weak to do so. That's why it's important for all of us to keep our muscles strong—something that even the elderly can work on.

Of course, conventional doctors often do recommend exercises and other forms of physical therapy to heal from musculoskeletal problems—although sometimes dismissively. Here's a story from my own experience. When I was twenty, I sprained my left ankle quite severely when my foot got caught between two railroad tracks. Although I did heal from the incident, it led to a cascade of other joint issues over the years, probably because my overall skeletal frame now had a weakness at a very important joint. As both chiropractors and osteopaths have reminded me over the years, the musculoskeletal system is one big interconnected mechanism. One weak link can propagate and affect many others, and often in not so obvious ways. Back when I was twenty, though, I knew nothing about chiropractic or osteopathy, and I didn't even get the help of physical therapy. The infirmary at my university simply recommended heat and ice and gave me an ace bandage and crutches to help me hobble around campus for a couple of weeks.

Unfortunately, by the time I was in my late 50s, I started having recurring issues with my ankle. It would lock, flare up with pain and swelling, and I'd sometimes have to use an ankle brace and cane for a week. Over time, these incidents became more frequent and long lasting. Finally I saw an orthopedic surgeon and got an MRI. He told me that my ankle ligament was stretched out after all these years and would continue to be problematic until I got surgery. When I asked about exercise therapy, he dismissively handed me a piece of paper with some illustrated exercises and assured me I'd be back for surgery soon.

Naturally, surgery isn't something I enjoy subjecting myself to. For one thing, I am sensitive to antibiotics and I didn't want to risk a hospital infection. I decided to seek out a physical therapist instead. Happily, after a couple of months of physical therapy, I was doing much better. Unlike most people, however, I decided to keep doing the recommended ankle exercises indefinitely. It's been many years now since I've been doing fifteen minutes of ankle exercises every day. I've only had a few incidents with my ankle since that time, and have always recovered nicely with continued exercise. For a few years I used an ankle brace when I took longer walks or hikes, but that is generally unnecessary now.

Posture Therapies

Most of us associate the word "posture" with our parents nagging us to "sit up straight!" or our gym teacher calling us to straight-backed attention. Because of this, cultivating good posture can seem like an annoyance and, in general, has become devalued and even mocked in today's world. But the truth is, the way we hold our bodies not only tells people a lot about our age, occupation, and sense of self-worth, but it also affects the health of our internal organs. In fact, poor posture is one of the primary causes of musculoskeletal pain. In a way, poor posture is a great example of not living in synchrony and alignment—with your physical structure.

Have you ever seen a photograph of people taken back in the 1800s? The way they sat and stood is completely different from how people hold their bodies today. I used to think this was due to cultural norms of formality associated with getting a photograph taken back then; after all, it was a unique and unusual event. But I have now learned that these photographs actually do depict the way people stood and sat in those days. Yes, women wore corsets, but men and children didn't. What's even more amazing is that the depiction in medical texts of a "normal spine" looks completely different today than it used to be. The average spine of today's modern person has become much more "S" shaped. Unfortunately, an exaggerated spinal curvature tends to increase with age in those with poor posture, and it can then lead to a lot of health problems.

How did this all happen? It turns out that fashion may have been the culprit. In the early 1900s, fashion models adopted a slouch in order to impart a feeling of freedom and nonchalance in their photos. Look at images of the flappers in the 1920s and you will notice it. Gone were the corsets and tight dresses. It was time to let it all hang out and slouch! Unfortunately, poor posture became equated with wealth, elegance, and sexual allure. Over the next 100 years, poor posture slowly became the norm.

If you sit in any café or restaurant and observe the patrons today, you will start to notice how bad most people's posture is. Now that I know better, it pains me to look! Even our chairs and car seats have been altered to accommodate our new postural habits. As we sit at our computers all day, we crane our necks forward. As we habitually look down at our cell phones, we create new and deeper postural pathologies. The habit of arching the back is another poor habit adopted by many young women in an attempt to appear more sexually attractive. When the increased curvature in our lower back pains us, we are told to "tuck in our butts" in order to straighten things out. Unfortunately, this only exacerbates problems further up the spine. Is there a better way? Fortunately, the answer is *yes*.

I first became aware of the critical importance of posture many years ago when I was taking voice lessons. In order to improve my breathing, my voice teacher recommended that I see a practitioner of the *Alexander Technique*. F.M. Alexander developed his posture therapy in the late 1800s and early 1900s and wrote his landmark book, *The Use of the Self*.[5] Many actors and musicians study the Alexander Technique in order to improve their stage presence and their ability to play instruments for long periods of time. If you pay attention, you may notice that many (but not all) actors have excellent posture.

My posture awareness became even more piqued, however, when I took the six-lesson sequence of the *Gokhale Method*, a therapy that I truly recommend to everyone. In fact, it should be taught in every elementary school. Posture pioneer Esther Gokhale[4] made an important discovery: the solution to today's posture problems can be found by observing the postural habits of people who weren't influenced by the slouching trends of the 1900s. She spent decades studying and photographing people living in indigenous or non-Westernized societies. After closely observing the way they stand, sit, sleep, walk, lift, and bend, she understood that there is indeed a reason why even the very elderly in those societies are able to endure hours of picking crops in the fields; they know how to use their bodies correctly. They have not forgotten the postures and movements that were perfected over a million years of human evolution. So, the musculoskeletal pain and poor breathing experienced by even young people today are a modern phenomenon. Happily, we can unlearn bad postural habits and regain our natural human posture with just a little bit of effort. The Gokhale Method is one way to do so. Using Esther Gokhale's images as an instructional tool, her posture lessons instruct students, in a hands-on way, how to properly sit, stand, walk, sleep, and bend. I can attest that this information has been life-transforming for me and other members of my family.

My journey to the Gokhale Method began when I was in my late 50s. I had begun to experience occasional tingling on the right side of my face, right arm, and right leg. Of course, I was worried. I went to my allopathic doctor fearing the worst, but she assured me that my symptoms were not due to a neurological disease. Next came a visit to my osteopath, who told me that my jaw was the culprit—and it is true that I have a very poor bite, grind my teeth, and suffered from occasional bouts of jaw locking. I also tend to have a forward neck posture. The osteopath then sent me to a dentist who specializes in temporomandibular joint (TMJ) disorders. Rather than treating me with an appliance, however, he told me that my real problem was that I was a lifelong mouth breather and tongue-thruster—that is, I didn't swallow properly, thrusting my tongue forward instead of upward and backward. So, my journey continued when I was sent to an orofacial myofunctional therapist who specializes in correcting this problem.[6]

After six months of working on becoming a nose breather and learning to swallow properly, I had gained a great deal. My therapist was wonderful and taught me that my poor bite, jaw issues, and forward neck posture were due to almost 60 years of poor breathing and swallowing. Despite the fact that I was one of her oldest patients (most were about 8 years old!), I did make great progress. But I still felt occasional tingling on the right side of my body. She told me that although my underlying issues had been mostly corrected, I still had to work on my neck posture. As it turns out, if you're a mouth breather and tongue-thruster, you actually *need* to hold your neck forward in order to breathe. Over the years, my forward neck posture had become pronounced enough that it affected the nerves in my neck—hence the tingling.

My final stop on this journey was Esther Gokhale and her posture therapy. Happily, after six weeks of lessons, the tingling ended! It still comes up a bit if I'm tense or under stress, but if I correct my neck posture and relax, it goes away. I also notice that when I sit, stand, and walk correctly, I literally look ten years younger. Now that's something we would all like for ourselves! And here's one amusing end to this story. Imagine my surprise when I opened up Esther Gokhale's wonderful book, *8 Steps to a Pain Free Back*,[7] and found that the Forward had been written by my allopathic physician! My voyage had gone full circle.

If I have inspired you to improve your health by addressing your posture, a good place to begin is to find an Alexander teacher, or perhaps even better, a Gokhale Method teacher. Both are international organizations. Esther Gokhale is also beginning to branch out into online teaching. While reading books and watching videos can be very helpful, however, nothing can replace being guided by someone else's hands so that you can discover what good posture actually feels like in your Physical Body.

Movement Therapies and Massage

Another way of improving how you hold and use your body is to engage in one of many possible movement therapies. These therapies usually entail taking a class of some kind and then regularly practicing the recommended movements. Included in this category are Yoga,

Feldenkrais, Pilates, Qi Gong, and Tai Chi. Of course, there are many more such therapies—every culture has its own to offer.

The idea behind movement therapies is that they increase body awareness and strengthen certain muscles, and in so doing, improve posture, breathing, and a sense of well-being. In essence, they help you to live in synchrony with your physical frame. Many are also based on the structures of the Etheric Body and can thus be viewed as etherically-based therapies too. This is certainly true of Yoga, Qi Gong, and Tai Chi, as well as many martial arts.

While movement therapies require you to move in order to become aware of your Physical Body, another approach is to have someone else help you do so. That's the idea behind massage. Of course, most of us are familiar with massage as a way of relaxing muscles through external touch, pressure, and kneading by a practitioner. Some massage techniques also incorporate the use of hot stones or the use of aromatic oils that can affect the emotions.

But many varieties of massage go way beyond relaxation. Some are focused on literally restructuring your musculature (for example, Rolfing) or intensively releasing muscular knots (Myofascial Trigger Point Therapy). Others use pressure to massage internal organs—especially the gut (Visceral Massage). Then there are Shiatsu, Trager, Reflexology, and so many other options. Ayurveda and Chinese medicine also recommend various types of massage. Indeed, every culture has its own practices, many of which are guided by the architecture of the Etheric Body.

To investigate a particular movement therapy or massage technique, your best bet is to use the internet to learn more and find a recommended class or practitioner. Know that not all methodologies are suitable for everyone, and that some can be quite intense. Also know that engaging in a movement technique can, at times, evoke releases within the energy bodies or trigger cleansing reactions like fatigue and detoxification. I remember how one visceral massage session left me tired for hours. I have also found that receiving a standard deep tissue massage can sometimes trigger a cleansing cold, which releases mucus from the body.

Of course, you will probably only know if something is for you if you try it. Use your intuition. See if it helps you and perhaps more importantly, if you enjoy it. Also resist the temptation to believe that a particular method or technique is *the* answer for all your problems. While a particular movement therapy might be helpful to you, it may also be true that the root of a particular problem lies not in your Physical Body, but in one of your higher energy bodies.

Chiropractic and Osteopathy

I have already mentioned Ayurveda and Chinese medicine as forms of holistic medicine that view the Physical Body as an interconnected system governed by the Etheric Body. Such practitioners understand that the body is inherently self-healing and provide treatments that foster this innate power. Two other holistic systems of medicine are Chiropractic and Osteopathy. Practitioners of these healing arts also see the body as an interconnected whole that is self-healing and connected to a vital, energetic, Etheric Body. However, their primary method of healing is through external manipulation of the Physical Body. In essence, they use their hands to help you to physically "line up."

Of these two systems, chiropractic is probably the one most familiar to you, being very common in the West. Chiropractors study at four-year schools and earn a degree that gives them the title Doctor of Chiropractic (DC). They are licensed by the government in most places. While their training includes the basics of overall medicine, a chiropractor's primary focus is on the musculoskeletal system. Indeed, most people go to a chiropractor because they are dealing with aches and pains that seem to originate in their bones, muscles, tendons, ligaments, etc. Nevertheless, the underlying philosophy of chiropractic stresses that the entire human being is an interconnected whole. Thus, many other kinds of ailments can be affected and healed by chiropractic treatment too.

Chiropractors are also trained to use other modalities, not just physical adjustments. They often give dietary advice or dispense supplements and sometimes dispense homeopathic remedies. One chiropractor I know prescribes specific exercises as his primary tool, at least whenever possible. Nevertheless, the main focus of chiropractic practice is on spinal adjustment.

Anyone who has been to a chiropractor knows the routine and remembers the experience well—receiving that neck or back "crack" that can bring a sense of relief. The reasoning behind a chiropractic adjustment is that many bodily dysfunctions are rooted in spinal *subluxations*—points of poor alignment in the spine's vertebrae. The goal of an adjustment is to correct them. Indeed, chiropractors believe that a subluxation, even if slight, can potentially affect many parts of the body. The founder of chiropractic, Daniel David Palmer (1845-1913), felt that although various forms of manipulation had been used for healing for thousands of years, no one had developed a scientific rationale to explain their efficacy. Once he developed the principle of subluxation and refined his adjustment technique, he found that he was able to cure many more people.

One form of chiropractic care that I have recently become a fan of is Zone Chiropractic.[8] Rather than focusing on "cracking" the back or neck, this system divides the spine into six zones, each of which affects different organ systems. Each treatment begins with a technique to determine which zone to work on. Then, an adjustment primarily utilizes various tools to stimulate those regions of the spine. Although a Zone Chiropractic treatment session is typically quite brief, I can attest to the fact that it can have profound effects.

Like chiropractors, osteopaths are also holistically trained. However, osteopathic medical schools are much more like conventional allopathic medical schools. Osteopaths attend four-year programs that cover essentially the same material as conventional medical schools and they even enter into hospital residencies. After graduation, they earn the title Doctor of Osteopathy (DO) and are licensed and accepted as fully functioning medical doctors with hospital privileges. However, unlike in conventional medicine, osteopathy places more stress on the interconnectedness of the Physical Body and its inherent ability to heal. It also recognizes the existence of the vital energy body—the Etheric Body.

One aspect of traditional osteopathic training is the use of hands-on manipulation. In recent times, however, most DOs have begun to function more like MDs and do not train extensively in hands-on techniques nor utilize them in their practices. So, if you would like to see an osteopath for osteopathic manipulation, you should first determine if they are primarily focused on this in their practice.

I usually call hands-on osteopathy "traditional osteopathy," because it was osteopathic manipulation that was the primary contribution and focus of osteopathy's founder, Andrew Taylor Still (1828-1917). Like Palmer, Still realized that disease could originate in slight anatomical deviations, so he developed techniques to correct them. Unlike Palmer, however, Still was an allopath who added manipulation to his conventional practice. Over time, this led to the more conventional nature of osteopathic training.

Going to a traditional osteopath is actually quite different than a chiropractic visit. Unlike a chiropractic adjustment, osteopathic treatment is gentler, subtler, and sometimes imperceptible. You can even fall asleep on an osteopath's treatment table! You might think of the process as gently guiding and providing information to the body so that it can correct itself. There is also a focus on aligning the cranial bones and sacrum (pelvic area) in order to alleviate compression and free up movement of cerebrospinal fluid. One form of massage, Craniosacral Massage, also has this goal, although its practitioners are usually massage therapists who take a few classes in the method. In contrast, hands-on traditional osteopaths have spent years perfecting their technique.

Although this kind of osteopathy is quite subtle, it can be transformational. I've personally experienced it and witnessed its beneficial effects on several family members and friends.

Finally, I'll conclude with a piece of advice I mentioned at the beginning of this chapter. Many practitioners, from herbalists to chiropractors, want their patients to continue visiting them for ongoing long-term treatment, often weekly. In my view, this might indicate that their treatment, though alleviating, may not be curative. This means that you should also look elsewhere for answers. In my experience, these answers will likely be found at energetic levels of your being—in your Etheric, Astral, Mental, or Causal Body.

CHAPTER 15

❧

WE ARE BEINGS GOVERNED BY ENERGY AND VIBRATION

Every system of medicine that I am aware of—except one—acknowledges a fundamental aspect of our true nature: *we are more than our physical bodies*. These systems recognize that an invisible energetic force interpenetrates our being and that it ultimately governs how our body functions. This force and its energy go by many names, depending on language and culture: *chi* (also written as *qi* or *ki*), *shakti*, *prana*, *vital force*, *manna*, *od*, and more. In this book, I refer to the body's vital force as the *Etheric Body*, a term used by esoteric teacher Rudolf Steiner, among many others. And because of the primacy of the Etheric Body in maintaining our health, perhaps the most powerful way to heal on the physical level is to tune its etheric energy in some way.

How ironic it is that the only outlier among world medicines on this subject is modern allopathic medicine! Perhaps in its eagerness to adopt a completely materialistic and mechanistic view of reality—a view that admittedly has also yielded vast knowledge and power over the physical—modern medicine has thrown the baby out with the bathwater. As a result, allopathy has limited and disempowered itself, condemning so many people to a bleak and unhealthy future— one in which humans are seen as no more than biological robots, composed of cells and organs, pipes and conduits, through which chemicals flow.

Luckily, other healing systems are still going strong and curing people all over the world. Despite the fact that allopathic medicine and its beneficiaries and promoters, the pharmaceutical and insurance industries, have amassed immense financial and political power, the so-called "alternative" systems of healing continue to be popular. Why? Because they work. They are also usually more affordable and accessible and can create more long-lasting good health and happiness. Thank goodness! Because the cracks in the allopathic edifice are growing larger every day. I believe that the failures surrounding the COVID era will only exacerbate this trend—if these failures are acknowledged and not censored from our awareness.

While allopathy is still largely operating on the mechanistic premises of the 1800s and has barely begun to admit 20th and 21st century revelations about quantum physics into its world-view, out on the margins, frontier scientists are beginning to prove the existence of the human energy body. Perhaps it will take another 100 years, but eventually, the Etheric Body—the fundamental lattice upon which our Physical Body is built and the ultimate governor of its shape and function—will be recognized and incorporated into *all* forms of medicine.

Healing systems that acknowledge the Etheric Body tend to have a different view about what creates health and disease—a view that is fundamentally *holistic*. They see each patient as a unique and united (whole) system of functioning—one in which physical symptoms, emotions, thoughts, and behaviors are inextricably interconnected and interdependent. Disease is not viewed as an external entity to be banished or a plumbing problem to be manually fixed, but rather, as an overall state of being within each individual patient. Treatment then proceeds from this holistic premise. Symptoms are understood as signposts of the greater whole, not as pests to be eradicated and suppressed. And once a practitioner understands a patient's holistic state of "dis-ease," treatment can be applied to help shift their state to a healthier one.

Holistic systems also recognize the whole-body nature of the healing process itself. For example, they understand that with successful treatment, not just a single symptom will improve, but many other things will begin to heal as well. Sleep, excretion, and emotional state may all improve along with a patient's primary physical complaint. Other common symptoms of true healing include a discharge of toxins, a return of older long-suppressed symptoms, and sometimes other mysterious reactions, all initiated by the inscrutable but wise Etheric Body. No matter what the holistic system of healing may be, there is also a recognition that it is not the practitioner's intervention that is truly doing the healing, but rather, the Etheric Body itself. That is, a practitioner is *triggering the inherent self-healing and self-regulating abilities of the Etheric Body, and then, by extension, the healing of the Physical Body*. In contrast, allopathic interventions usually attempt to force some kind of change upon the Physical Body.

If you think about it, there is a logical reason why an acknowledgement of the Etheric Body leads to the holistic viewpoint. If an etheric energy does pervade our entire being, it can't be limited to one organ system or body part. Although some etherically-based healing systems (notably acupuncture) do utilize structural models of the Etheric Body to guide treatment, every etherically-oriented system of medicine recognizes that the activity of the Etheric Body is ultimately mysterious and operates according to its own logic.

To summarize, the Etheric Body is a whole and powerful system in its own right, with rules, mechanisms, and strategic choices of its own. It is our piece of a much larger, interconnected, and mysterious etheric puzzle. It is also our most far-reaching locus of healing because the Etheric Body not only controls our Physical Body, but also provides the primary connection to our higher energy bodies. For this reason, healing at the etheric level can help to heal our Astral, Mental, and Causal Bodies too.

The rest of this chapter focuses on etherically-focused healing modalities. Some do not use any direct physical intervention at all, but instead, rely on the fact that some form of healing energy will, nevertheless, enter the patient's Etheric Body and do its work. For example, this is true of Reiki, crystal healing, and sound healing. Other etheric modalities do use physical interventions that penetrate, touch, or move the body in some way, but are directed toward the etheric level. This is true of homeopathy, acupuncture, acupressure, and Qi Gong. Although etherically-focused practitioners may utilize pills, liquids, needles, or movements, they know that what they are actually achieving is not fundamentally chemical or physical in nature.

SIGNS AND CAUTIONS FOR THE ETHERIC REALM

Let's begin by considering signs that an ailment is rooted in the Etheric Body.

Signs that your problem may be etherically based

The number one indication that a physical problem is actually rooted in the Etheric Body is that it is chronic. In other words, all helpful physical treatments are simply palliative (they only alleviate things for a while) or are suppressive (they act only by masking symptoms, which then likely reappear elsewhere, often in a deeper and more chronic form).

Unfortunately, chronic disease is rampant in our society today. Very often, this is due to suppressive treatment. Examples include systemic issues like eczema, allergies, chronic or recurring infections (including bacterial, viral, and parasitical infections), gastrointestinal problems, headaches, neurological disorders, and cancer. Unlike allopathic treatments, etheric modalities can sometimes completely cure these problems. They can also speed the healing of problems that *are* more physical in nature, including epidemic diseases, broken bones, toxic exposures, and problems that arise from surgery, chemotherapy, or radiation. Because etheric healing can also reach into the emotional and mental realms, it can be successful in treating emotional and mental problems too.

Personally, I have found that etheric modalities are particularly useful when a doctor has no idea what's wrong or what to do about it. When an allopath doesn't have a "diagnosis," they simply can't prescribe. In contrast, etheric healers generally treat based on the symptoms being experienced and trust in the wisdom of the Etheric Body to heal itself. For example, even in a virulent epidemic, a homeopath just needs to know your symptoms in order to select an effective remedy; a diagnosis, test, or the identification of a pathogen is not necessary at all.

Etheric modalities are also useful if you suspect a problem has arisen due to some mysterious external cause that isn't readily apparent. Because the Etheric Body isn't physically compartmentalized and is linked to the general etheric realm, it interacts freely with the energies of other people, plants, and animals without you realizing it. As a result, you may mysteriously develop the symptoms of other family members, even if they aren't supposedly contagious.

Interestingly, some people have suggested that infectious diseases aren't really transmitted by physical "germs" at all, but rather, by some form of etheric contagion that germs are attracted to. Though germs may be present, they are just going along for the ride. If this is true, it could explain why some people are susceptible to a particular disease while others are not; their Etheric Bodies are different. For example, I have found that I am much less susceptible to colds and flus ever since I started homeopathic treatment. Maybe it's because my physical immune system was strengthened. Or maybe it's because my etheric boundaries are now less permeable.

Another indicator of an etheric problem is if an issue with the electromagnetic spectrum is suspected. This is because the Etheric Body is highly interactive with EMFs (electromagnetic fields). For example, electromagnetic sensitivities or the occurrence of mysterious breakages in electronic devices in your home might point to personal problems on the etheric level.

Moreover, even when the actual root of a particular health problem lies in an even higher energy body, especially in the Astral Body, it may still manifest as abnormalities in the Etheric Body, which then interacts with EMFs. Anyone who has worked in an office setting knows how computer systems tend to fail when tensions are flaring. Here is a story illustrating this phenomenon that was experienced by my husband Steve. The whole episode occurred soon after he took a homeopathic remedy—an etheric level intervention.

At the time when all of this occurred, Steve was experiencing some troublesome physical symptoms and was also quite unhappy at work. He saw our homeopath and she prescribed a remedy that, no doubt, took all of these factors into account. A couple of weeks later, as he was driving home from work, Steve's car stereo system stopped working. Upon sitting at his home computer, he then discovered that his keyboard was no longer functioning. Shortly thereafter, his computer crashed too—a complete hard drive failure. This was a true cascade of electronic malfunction! To add something even more mysterious into the mix, the name of the computer program that Steve was busy developing (and had been working on for over 30 years) was "Electric."

Completely furious at this point, Steve drove off to buy a new hard drive. Both of us have doctorates in computer science and Steve is truly a pro at fixing these kinds of problems. Nevertheless, even after he swapped keyboards, installed a new hard drive, and began to rebuild his operating system, he simply could not get his computer to work. In fact, he banged his head against the problem for over a week. I kept telling Steve that the issue wasn't his computer at all—it was within him. His etheric energy was in such turmoil that it was causing all of his personal electronic devices to break.

Eventually, Steve decided to stay up all night and keep working on his computer. During that time, he did a lot of soul searching and made a major decision about cutting back his hours at work and ultimately retiring. Within minutes, his computer began to function normally. The next day, when he got into his car, the stereo was working perfectly, despite the fact that he had done nothing to repair it. His physical problems subsequently got much better too.

What's the moral of this story? The thoughts and feelings of the Mental and Astral Bodies directly interact with the Etheric and Physical Bodies, which also interact with the energies of the environment. It's all one big stew. And if you want to live in synchrony with it all, you need to work at *all* levels.

Signs that the problem is not just etheric and might be helped by astral, mental, or causal approaches:

What if both physical and etheric interventions are only palliative and help only for a short while? Or what if they must be utilized repeatedly over long periods of time? This is a sign that the root of the problem may lie even deeper. While etheric treatments are usually not suppressive like allopathic medicines, they still can be insufficient to do the trick. That's when you need to dig even deeper and address problems in the higher energy bodies, especially the Astral Body (the subject of Chapter 16)— just like Steve did when he realized how unhappy he was and that he needed to make some real changes in his life. If a problem occurred directly after an emotional event or trauma, or appeared during significant life changes like retirement, divorce, prolonged care-giving for a loved one, or a death or birth in the family, astral level healing might be the answer.

Cautions for etheric-level treatment:

Just as I mentioned in Chapter 14, my first word of advice when selecting a therapy or therapist is to trust your instincts, intuitions, and sensations. If you suspect that a therapy or practitioner is not for you, discontinue it.

Next, *do not assume that because etherically-based treatment is not physical in nature, it is innocuous. It is not.* Such therapies can be just as powerful as physically-based treatments, often even more so! Do not pop homeopathic remedies willy-nilly. Also be circumspect about your use of sound therapies and crystals. And do not see a hands-on energy healer if you suspect that *their* energy might be unhealthy or unstable.

Just as for a conventional doctor, some form of practitioner certification is always preferable and recommendations are always helpful. Because most issues addressed by etheric-level practitioners tend to be chronic in nature, you will likely be seeing them regularly, at least for a while. That is why your relationship with them must be comfortable. And be patient! Do not expect the first treatment or intervention to mysteriously work and cure you. If an allopath hasn't been able to help you, why should a homeopath, acupuncturist, or hands-on healer be able to instantly and magically cure you? Usually, several follow-up trips to the practitioner are needed so that treatments can be adjusted or modified over time.

Finally, educate yourself about the nature of etherically-based healing sensations and processes. Healing at this level simply does not feel the same as taking a pharmaceutical drug. In fact, you may not notice anything consciously at all but just mysteriously feel better. When that happens, you might even attribute it to something else. On the other hand, if you are sensitive, you might initially experience sensations like tingling and energy flows.

Also be cognizant of the fact that successful etheric healing can trigger a variety of phenomena that are signs of the Etheric Body in action. All of the following phenomena, mysterious though they may be, can be considered positive signs of healing at the etheric level:

- Temporary aggravation of symptoms.

- The release of discharges like mucus or diarrhea for a few days, or even some vomiting or a cold or flu.

- Emotions that have been bottled up are released and aggravated for a while.

- Old symptoms that had been suppressed return. Often these symptoms will fade on their own, but sometimes they may require further treatment. Many practitioners refer to this phenomenon as "peeling the onion." That is, recent problems are cured, but former ones must now be addressed.

Etherically-Based Therapies

Now let's consider a variety of etheric-level therapies individually. Obviously, there are many more that I could talk about; I'm presenting only a representative sampling that I am personally familiar with. I have categorized them into two broad categories: ones that utilize some form of physical intervention or application that inserts something into the body, and ones that do not.

Approaches that access the Etheric Body through physical interventions that insert something into the body:

- Homeopathy

- Traditional Chinese Medicine (TCM) (e.g., acupuncture)

Approaches that access the Etheric Body only through touch, movement, or external energies:

- Hands-on healing (Barbara Brennan healing, Reiki, Quantum Touch)

- Energy exercises like Yoga, Tai Chi, and Qi Gong

- Sound therapies

- Healing with crystals and geometry

- Muscle Testing (applied kinesiology)

Approaches that access the Etheric Body through physical interventions that insert something into the body

Homeopathy

By this point, you probably realize that homeopathy is the therapy I know the best. In fact, I wrote a whole introductory book about it! So please forgive me for writing more about this form of medicine than I do others. Homeopathy is my family's go-to medicine of choice and has worked many miracles in our lives, the biggest miracle of all being our very first. When my younger son Max was three years old and my husband and I were both computer science researchers in Silicon Valley, we learned about homeopathy as a possible treatment for his growing behavioral and language issues—problems that have now become familiar to too many parents all over the world: autism. In our case, this was way back in early 1995, at the very beginning of the autism explosion.

The healing we witnessed in our son Max was nothing short of miraculous. Within a week of giving him the prescribed homeopathic remedy, we noticed subtle changes that were also noted by his therapist (even though we did not tell her about this new intervention). After three months, the improvements in his language and behavior could not be denied. In less than a year, Max's therapist decided that her treatments were no longer needed. After 18 months, we signed papers releasing him from eligibility for special education benefits. For those interested in learning more about homeopathy than I am able to present in this book (including the story of Max's cure and other people's amazing cure stories for a wide variety of ailments), check out my book *Impossible Cure*.[1]

Naturally, Max's recovery was a mind-blowing experience for our entire family. We all began to see a homeopath and experienced more remarkable healings. Although Steve and I were scientists and had always been wedded to allopathy (in fact, Steve's father was an allopath), we couldn't deny that homeopathy's ultradilute remedies were somehow acting upon an unseen part of us. Eventually, I began to study homeopathy formally, decided to write a book to let more people know about it, and became active in the homeopathic community, including political work to ensure its legal practice. Ever since that time, our lives have been slowly transformed by events that began in 1995.

So what *is* homeopathy? If you are currently unfamiliar with this modality, the first thing to know is that the term "homeopathy" is usually misused by the media and in colloquial speech. "Homeopathy" is *not* a general term for natural or holistic medicine and it has nothing to do with diets, herbs, or supplements. Instead, its essence is defined by its name. "Homeo" means *similar* and "pathy" means *suffering*. More specifically, homeopathy is a system of medicine based on a single underlying principle of practice and law of nature called the "Law of Similars." It can be stated as follows:

> *If a substance is capable of creating symptoms in a healthy person that are similar to those that a patient is experiencing, it can be prepared and applied in such a way that it cures the patient.*

In other words, the curative medicine for each patient is the one that causes *similar suffering*—i.e., is *homeo-pathic* to the patient.

One way that I like to illustrate this principle is with the use of coffee. Coffee affects us in profound ways and that's why we like to drink it. It produces many emotional, mental, and physical effects, including a sense of elation, intensified mental focus, and sometimes heart palpitations and activation of the bowels. It's similar to the state you might experience after a fun night partying and can't get to sleep. This kind of insomnia has many of the same characteristics as the "coffee state": elation, a mind full of thoughts, palpitations, and active bowels. And that's why it can be treated by the homeopathic remedy made from coffee—*Coffea*.

Now let me quickly make two important points. Notice that I used the phrase "remedy made from coffee." Drinking a cup of coffee before bed is not a good way to fall asleep! While the Law of Similars *can* work if a substance is used in its crude form (think about how allopaths use the stimulant Ritalin to calm down speedy hyperactive children—a practice that unwittingly utilizes the power of the Law of Similars), homeopathic remedies are almost always prepared so that the physical substance from which they are made is removed—leaving behind only its *energy* or *vibration*. Although this energy is typically transmitted to a patient via pills or liquids, it is *not* operating through chemical means. How so? Because the remedy preparation process renders it chemically inert from a materialistic viewpoint. That is why homeopathy is an etherically-based form of medicine. It is also why it has been controversial ever since its development over 200 years ago.

The second important point is that, unlike in allopathy, there is typically no "take this for that" approach in homeopathic practice. Insomnia, for instance, can take many forms. Sometimes it arises due to anger, anxiety, or grief. Sometimes it wakes us up in the middle of the night rather than keeping us awake at bedtime. These other types of insomnia would not call for Coffea Cruda, but rather, a different remedy—one with its own matching insomnia symptoms. In fact, there are many commonly used insomnia remedies.

Not surprisingly, homeopathy has always been controversial to materialistic scientists. Fifty years ago, it was marginalized, largely ignored by the media, and homeopaths were generally left to practice in peace. Today, pharmaceutical companies are investing a lot of money to launch media and political attacks on homeopathy—and most recently, trying to limit public access to homeopathic remedies.[2] Why? You might think it's about financial competition (which is actually negligible compared to the financial power of pharmaceutical companies). Personally, I think it's because science is beginning to verify the power of homeopathy's energy-extraction process. The pharmaceutical companies may actually be realizing that the same process can be used to extract the energy-signature of *all* drugs.[3] If this information became widely accepted, the cost of allopathic drugs would plummet. More on this later.

So how was this mysterious energy-extraction technique developed?

In the late 1700s, Dr. Samuel Hahnemann, the developer of homeopathy, was a respected young doctor in Germany. Steeped in the growing interest in science during that time period, as well as in the importance of critically observing patients, Hahnemann became alarmed by the crude methods of his peers—practices like bloodletting and the administration of toxic substances like mercury. He began to realize that these methods were, in fact, doing more harm than good. Eventually, he wrote widely-read, scathing papers explaining his views, gave up the traditional practice of medicine, and turned to chemistry and medical translation as a way to support his family.

One day, Hahnemann was translating a text about the curative powers of a new and effective medicine for malaria made from a tree bark: quinine. He decided to conduct an experiment upon himself and discovered that when he took quinine, he developed, for a few hours, the same fever and rigors that are characteristic of malaria. In a stroke of insight, he realized that this new drug was able to cure malaria because it could cause its symptoms! Based on this observation, Hahnemann developed the principle of *homeo-pathy* (an idea also mentioned by Hippocrates) and began testing it and writing about it. An interesting side note: it was Hahnemann who first coined the term "allopathy," because the word "allo" means "other" in contrast to "homeo" meaning similar.

Over time, Hahnemann gained many followers of his new theory within the medical community. In the early 1800s, he was able to successfully treat several virulent epidemics that other doctors had no success with—for example, the typhoid fever epidemic of 1813. As a result, Hahnemann's fame began to grow and spread all over Europe, and an increasing number of doctors world-wide began to abandon allopathy for homeopathy. Not surprisingly, this led to the first political attacks on homeopathy by allopathic doctors in both Europe and America.

Of course, because Hahnemann was also a chemist, he realized that giving toxic substances to his patients was not a great idea, even if they were technically homeopathic. So he began to dilute them in an effort to reduce their toxicity. Unfortunately, they stopped working when he did so. In his next effort, Hahnemann began to shake the remedy solutions vigorously between each dilution step in order to make sure that they were thoroughly mixed. Amazingly, they began to work again! In fact, he discovered that the more the remedies were diluted and shaken, the less toxic they became and the more curatively they acted.

Hahnemann called this new method of remedy preparation *potentization*, because he realized that although there was likely not a single particle of the original substance in them, they *did* contain a potent power that must have been latent in the substance to begin with. He even discovered that normally benign and nonmedicinal substances like salt or other minerals could become curative once they were potentized.

Next, in order to discover which ailments his remedies could treat, Hahnemann enlisted his growing coterie of likeminded doctors to subject themselves to homeopathic drug tests that he called *provings*. After they took the potentized substances, these doctors recorded their physical, emotional, mental, and behavioral symptoms over the next few weeks. These symptoms, along with symptom information culled from successful cures, were then compiled into books called *materia medica*. These became the medical reference books for homeopathic treatment. Interestingly, the same remedies and symptoms compiled in the 1800s are still used today because they are still valid. They simply state which symptoms a substance can cause, and therefore, what it can cure.

Now keep in mind, Hahnemann did most of this work in the early 1800s; he died in 1843. There was no scientific way to test what was going on within homeopathic remedies back then. Still, allopaths ridiculed homeopaths because their remedies were so dilute. Homeopathy was especially despised by the apothecaries (pharmacies) of that time because homeopaths usually manufactured their own remedies, which were also quite low in cost. Despite all of this, homeopathy spread all over the world during the remainder of the 1800s.

In America, for example, homeopathy's popularity grew because of its success in treating a wide variety of epidemics, including yellow fever. Homeopathy also became the medicine of choice for the cultural elite, for presidents, and for pioneers who carried homeopathic remedy kits as they travelled across the expanding nation. In fact, many of today's American medical schools began as homeopathic schools. In the meantime, the British brought homeopathy with them to the Indian subcontinent. Today, India is an important epicenter of homeopathy, with an entire system of fully accepted homeopathic medical schools. Homeopathy is also integrated into the health care systems of many European countries and in Latin America, with most of its practitioners being medical doctors.

Unfortunately, homeopathy's growing popularity made it a prime target for allopaths and their increasingly powerful ally, the pharmaceutical industry. This was especially true in the US. During the 1800s, doctors were banned from medical societies if they had anything to do with homeopathy or homeopaths. Indeed, the American Medical

Association was founded for this express purpose. After World War I, American homeopathic medical schools, along with the medical schools of other types of therapies, were gradually shut down or converted to allopathy. Homeopathy (and alternative medicine in general) went into a decline as a result. Luckily, it began to revive again in the 1970s when young medical students, steeped in the counter-culture movement, rediscovered it. With their growing successes (and allopathy's growing failures), homeopathy and other alternative healing modalities began to flourish once again.

Today, some fearless scientists are finally beginning to discover what makes homeopathic remedies work. For example, they have discovered that nanoparticles of the original substance may still be present in remedy dilutions. At the same time, water scientists have discovered that the homeopathic potentization process affects a dilution's water structure in measurable ways. And there is even some proof that it really may be *etheric energy* or *information* that is captured by potentization. For example, studies have demonstrated that the electromagnetic signature embedded in an ultradilution can be recorded, transmitted electronically, replayed into another vial of water in an entirely different location, and still have the same effects.[4]

So, what *is* the nature of this remedy signature? It's a vibration, a resonance. In essence, potentization extracts the "vibe" of a substance. Then, when a prover takes a potentized remedy to test its effects, they take on this vibration and the symptoms they develop reflect how this vibration plays out in their body. Since homeopathy's curative action occurs when a remedy's vibration is *similar* to ("homeopathic" to) the vibration of a patient, *it is literally the form of medicine that heals through the process of synchrony*. Homeopathy is *healing* in synchrony!

Now consider this. If a substance (including any allopathic drug) can be processed in such a way that its energetic signature can be recorded, emailed to you, and replayed into water, then *all* drugs, whether homeopathic or allopathic, would essentially become *free*. I believe this is why the pharmaceutical companies will do anything they can to suppress this information. Even Nobel-prize winning scientists have had their research banned when they studied this phenomenon. Consider what happened to Dr. Luc Montagnier, the French doctor who won the Nobel prize for discovering the relationship between AIDS and the HIV virus. When Montagnier discovered that ultradilutions of DNA still preserved the properties of the original DNA,[3] he lost all funding in Europe and was forced to relocate his research lab to China. Sadly, Dr. Montagnier died in 2022, but not until after he warned the world about the long-term dangers of the COVID-19 vaccine.

Before I conclude my discussion of homeopathy, there are a few points I'd like you to keep in mind if you decide to embark upon homeopathic treatment. Many of them apply to any form of holistic medicine.

First, *homeopathic treatment is based on the entire symptom complex of a patient—not just physical symptoms, but also emotional, mental, and behavioral symptoms.* Moreover, *this symptom complex is unique for each patient.* The process of homeopathic treatment is thus a two-step process: 1) find out what a patient's symptoms are; and 2) try to find the remedy whose symptoms best match it. In essence, it's all about finding a remedy that will "sync up" with a patient.

However, because of the vast scope of possible symptoms and the fact that there are nearly 2000 remedies, the homeopathic matching process is both highly analytical and artful in nature. Today, computer programs are employed to help narrow things down, with the "art" of homeopathy coming from practitioner experience and treatment strategies that have been developed over time. For example, just as in Ayurveda and Chinese medicine, homeopaths have discerned patient constitutional types and patterns that help to guide remedy selection. Nevertheless, it is often the case that several remedies must be tried before one that is truly helpful can be found.

Next, note that *no formal diagnosis is necessary for homeopathic treatment to proceed; only the symptoms are needed.* Moreover, *no matter what the diagnosis may be, homeopaths view each patient's individual experience of disease as unique.* This can be quite a boon when a disease or pathogen cannot be identified. But it can also mean that the treatment of even familiar diseases (like the flu) may take a bit more time. We all know that the flu's presentation each year can be different. But even in the same epidemic, one patient may react differently than another. This was particularly true of COVID. For this reason, there is no single remedy that's good for "flu" or any other disease, although there may be ten or so remedies that are commonly utilized for it. It is therefore the homeopath's job to figure out which remedy is right for each individual patient.

Another important aspect of homeopathic philosophy is its understanding of disease progression and what a true cure looks like. Over the past 200 years, homeopaths have realized that although an allopathic suppressive treatment may appear to be curative, it is often only masking disease symptoms and will eventually create even deeper problems down the line. That is why suppressed eczema can lead to asthma, and why suppressed arthritis can lead to heart disease.

The flip side of disease progression is what homeopaths call the *Law of Cure*—that is, what a true cure looks like. Homeopaths have observed that the vital force (i.e., the Etheric Body) usually heals the deepest and most serious problems first. As cure progresses, it then typically proceeds from the most recent problems to the oldest ones, from the innermost to the outermost of our beings, and from the torso and head outward to the limbs. While an acute disease may go through these steps quickly, a chronic disease may take some time to unwind, with careful changes in remedy and dosing required along the way.

Homeopaths also recognize that, despite the power of their etheric vibration-based remedies, patients live in a physical world with all of its many trials and tribulations. As a result, there is a limit to what remedies can accomplish if there are ongoing factors that maintain a disease state. Such factors include poor diet, an unhealthy dwelling place, the habitual and excessive use of drugs, and extreme emotional stressors. For this reason, it is also the job of the homeopath, as is true for all holistic practitioners, to investigate and provide advice about these other disease-promoting causes.

Finally, a key discovery that Hahnemann made—and one that is often not followed by many of today's homeopaths—is that *the less medicine given, the better.* Not only did he advise giving the minimal number of doses necessary to achieve a cure, but he also objected to mixing remedies together, since doing so creates confusion vis-à-vis their individual effects. Mixed remedies also make assessment of the curative process more difficult.

Unfortunately, Hahnemann's conservative approach to practice is often ignored by many homeopaths because it can be time-consuming, difficult, and requires lifelong study. It is much easier to revert to an allopathic "take this for that" mindset and hand out mixed formulas. It is also simpler to try to use some kind of device to select a remedy (a practice that, in my view, can be dubious) rather than to engage in a more careful analysis. One reason for these shortcuts is that many practitioners who utilize homeopathic remedies today (for example, chiropractors and some naturopaths) receive only minimal training in homeopathy during their education and are not equipped to engage in a deeper homeopathic analysis. For this reason, I usually recommend that homeopathic treatment be pursued with a practitioner who is primarily trained and focused on the use of homeopathy.

Traditional Chinese Medicine (TCM) (e.g., acupuncture)

Traditional Chinese Medicine (TCM) represents the healing wisdom of China, accumulated over thousands of years. Like Ayurveda, TCM incorporates the use of herbal remedies, massage, a diagnostic typology system based on physical, emotional, and behavioral characteristics, targeted dietary advice, and a recognition of the Etheric Body. In Ayurveda, the name of the etheric life-force energy is *prana*. In TCM, it is called *chi, qi,* or the Japanese form, *ki*. You are probably already familiar with these words, because it is incorporated into the names of several Asian movement therapies and martial arts like *Tai Chi, Qi Gong,* and *Aikido*. Tai Chi and Qi Gong, in particular, utilize a combination of body movements and postures, mental focus, and breathing techniques to improve the flow of qi in the body and thereby promote physical, emotional, and mental well-being.

Over the millennia, TCM has developed a detailed model of the Etheric Body and its relationship to physical organs and functions. In Ayurveda, the structure is simpler and focuses primarily on the *chakras*, energy vortices located along the central channel. To those who can see the etheric level, the chakras look like spinning wheels that bring etheric energy into and out of the Etheric Body. As I will discuss later, many hands-on approaches to etheric healing focus on the chakras, and there is a great deal of information about them online.

In TCM, the architecture of the Etheric Body is much more complex. In addition to the central channel, it includes many additional vertical lines of energy called *meridians*. These are like a road network of energetic flow within the Etheric Body. Each of the meridians is punctuated by dozens of points—locations that are the primary focus of *acupuncture*. Acupuncturists lightly insert very thin needles into these points in order to stimulate or increase etheric energy, unblock energy flow, or to remove excess built-up energy. Practices related to TCM also have the same goals. They include *acupressure* (the application of physical pressure or rubbing at the points), *moxibustion* (the burning of herbs above the skin at the acupuncture points), and *cupping* (the application of cups to the points, which exert a vacuum-like pull).

Because the etheric energy running through the meridians profoundly affects every aspect of our being, the etheric interventions of

TCM can be highly effective in treating the full spectrum of physical and emotional disease. Though it may seem like the insertion of needles, pressure, or heat are acting physically or neurologically, this is not the case. Just as homeopaths give physical pills or liquids that carry energy rather than chemicals, TCM techniques are physical interventions designed to affect the Etheric Body.

Of course, each system of medicine has its own philosophy about how the body works, what causes disease, and how cures take place. In homeopathy, treatment is guided by a patient's symptoms and application of the Law of Similars. In TCM, individualized patient diagnosis and treatment is also based on a variety of philosophical principles. One is that the human body can be viewed as a miniature version of the surrounding universe, and that smaller parts of the body reflect health in the body as a whole. In other words, "As above, so below; As below, so above." Because of this, TCM practitioners can influence a patient's organ systems by applying pressure or needles at certain points on the palm, sole of the foot, or ear, all of which are considered microcosms of the larger body. In other words, as in the palm of the hand, so in the rest of the Physical Body.

TCM also sees overall health as the result of harmony or disharmony between two opposing and complementary forces: *yin* and *yang*. These forces are also associated with the female/male dichotomy (yin being the receptive "female" energy and yang being the active "male" energy). Many of you are probably familiar with the yin/yang symbol: a circle divided by an "S" into light and dark sides. The light side of the circle represents yang and contains a small dark circle of yin in its center. The dark side of the circle represents yin and contains a small light circle of yang. These swirling shapes of dark and light represent the fact that there should always be a flow between yin and yang, with a hint of yin always emerging from within yang, and vice versa. Too much yang or too much yin is not good for our health.

The final grand philosophical component of TCM is its division of natural phenomena and the stages of life into five elements: *fire, earth, wood, metal,* and *water*. Each of these elements is associated with certain colors, body organs, senses, emotional states, and diseases. These elements are also considered to define the aspects or qualities of qi flowing along the meridians. Because each patient possesses a unique blend of the elements, TCM practice begins by first determining the nature of this blend (called the *Zheng* or pattern) and then applying TCM therapies (like acupuncture) to rebalance them.

Ever since the 1970s, the practice of TCM has spread throughout the Western world. It has been legalized and licensed in most states in the US, and there are schools that teach TCM in most metropolitan areas. Since there is no history of "bad blood" between allopathy and TCM (as there is between allopathy and homeopathy) and because it is seen as mysterious and foreign, practices like acupuncture have been more readily accepted by conventional medicine as an allied healing field.

Approaches that access the Etheric Body only through touch, movement, or external energies

So far, I have presented etheric healing techniques that require some form of direct intervention that inserts something into the body, usually with the help of a practitioner. But there are plenty of approaches that don't invade the body in any way. With a bit of knowledge, many of them can be done by you and applied either to yourself or to a friend or family member. Many of them simply use the hands. Others utilize sounds or crystals or geometric shapes. All are based on the idea that the etheric realm pervades all of physical reality and guides its functions. As a result, etheric energy in our hands or emanating from crystals can be used to heal. And since sound, like etheric energy, is essentially a vibration, it too can affect our well-being on all levels.

Hands-on Healing

Perhaps one of the most common forms of etheric healing is the "laying on of hands." Skeptics may say that any healing that occurs is due to the "placebo effect." Aside from the fact that placebo healing is probably the safest way to heal—certainly safer than pharmaceuticals—the truth is that the so-called placebo effect is utilized by *every* medical practitioner, including allopaths. In essence, it is healing at the astral, mental, or causal level.

I believe that hands-on healing generally operates through an actual transmission or manipulation of etheric energy—that is, it is an etheric form of healing. If you doubt its power is real, consider the fact that the healing of animals or even substances in laboratory test tubes has been shown to occur via the "laying on of hands." And if you'd like some proof that your own hands are permeated by etheric energy, simply perform the hand exercises described in Chapter 5. They will enable you to sense this energy for yourself.

As it turns out, my very first introduction to alternative medicine was in the form of hands-on healing. In the early 1980s, I was working as a computer science researcher at SRI International in Menlo Park, California. On my lunch breaks, I occasionally wandered over to a nearby metaphysical bookstore where I was drawn to two books by Barbara Brennan, *Hands of Light* and *Light Emerging*, bestsellers to this day.[5] I was fascinated by Brennan's drawings of the energy bodies and, especially, the kinds of energy-flow patterns she could see. Brennan described how these patterns were correlated with specific emotional states, coping mechanisms, personality types, and diseases. Her information added a whole new depth to my understanding of people and of my own inner feelings and perceptions when I interacted with them.

A few years later, in the early 1990s, I attended a weekend workshop taught by Brennan in San Francisco. Along with hundreds of other attendees, I was guided through exercises that taught us how to use our psychic powers to hold certain objects and find out something about their owners—a practice called *psychometry*. We were also instructed on how to sense objects at a distance with our "energy hands" and practice healing techniques. I had experiences that weekend that truly confirmed the reality of these phenomena for me.

Soon afterward, I had a few appointments with a Brennan-trained practitioner. Unlike some forms of hands-on healing, Barbara Brennan's techniques are applied with very specific goals in mind. They include sensing and correcting the rotational direction of the chakras, opening up closed chakras, and correcting the structure of chakras that are opened too wide or misshapen. Just as in acupuncture, this form of treatment has the goal of correcting the Etheric Body in a specific way.

There are also methods of hands-on healing that are less directed. Two of them are *Quantum Touch*[6] and *Healing Touch*,[7] both of which can be applied to others and oneself. They involve meditation, breathing, and knowledge of the chakra system, and utilize intuition to help detect problems within the Etheric Body. They then achieve healing by sending loving intent and creating resonance with it. All such methods are based on the idea that the Etheric Body will use this transmitted energetic information to heal itself in the best possible way.

Ironically, hands-on healing has had a better reception than other etheric therapies in conventional settings. My guess is that it's because it isn't taken very seriously by allopaths, who view it as inherently benign, much like a visit from a hospital chaplain. Healing Touch, in particular, has become very popular among nurses who gain certification and use it for patient healing in hospital settings.

Of course, there are many other forms of hands-on healing too. I'm sure every culture has its own variety. They include etheric healing techniques used by shamans in almost every country—for example, *Pranic Healing* (developed by a Chinese-Filipino spiritual teacher). The practice of *mesmerism* in Europe during the 1800s (in which practitioners swept their hands over an entranced subject and sometimes utilized magnets) could also be viewed as a form of hands-on etheric healing.

Finally, I'd like to discuss another hands-on healing technique that I have had some personal experience with—*Reiki*.[8] The Japanese word "Reiki" literally means divine (*rei*) energy (*ki*). My first experience with it was with the same practitioner I visited for Barbara Brennan-style healing. At one appointment, he told me about workshops he offered that delivered Reiki *attunements*, so I decided to attend two of them. What makes Reiki unique is that the practitioner is not seen as the one who is delivering etheric healing information to the recipient. Instead, the practitioner is viewed as a conduit for healing energies emanating from some other spiritual source. The Reiki attunements, as well as certain words and movements that initiate a Reiki session, are seen as "keys" that unlock this flow of energy. Once someone has received an attunement, they can invoke this energy and apply Reiki healing to themselves or others. Personally, I have found it to be helpful.

Energy Exercises

In this brief section, I'd like to mention several movement practices that, although they are typically seen as forms of physical exercise, are actually motivated by the structure of the Etheric Body. All originate in cultures that have traditionally embraced the reality of the etheric realm.

First is the Indian practice of *Yoga*. Today, Yoga classes are taught all over the world. Indeed, Yoga has become a veritable industry in the West and most people who go to Yoga classes view it as the latest trendy form of exercise. The truth is, however, that Yoga's growing popularity is actually testimony to its health-promoting power. It certainly does strengthen muscles and improves blood flow, breathing, posture, and peace of mind. But why does Yoga employ the particular exercises and breathing techniques that it does? Because they are rooted in the structure and function of the Etheric Body. That is why Yoga can help to heal every level of our being, from the physical up to the higher energy bodies too.

The same can be said of the traditional exercises and martial arts of China and Japan—most of which have the word "chi", "qi", or "ki" as part of their name. For instance, *Tai Chi*, like Yoga, involves very specific forms of movement. I took a Tai Chi class when I worked at NASA in the 1990s and I remember how complicated it was to learn even the short form. Tai Chi can be quite powerful and effective in promoting health and well-being because its movements help to energize the Etheric Body. Another movement therapy from China, *Qi Gong*, is a bit easier to perform and is more directly health-oriented in nature. I perform a 15-minute Qi Gong exercise every morning called Y-Dan, and I invariably feel more energized and happier afterward.[9]

It is also interesting to note that Yoga, Tai Chi, and Qi Gong movements are all accompanied by specific breathing patterns. That is because physical breath has an intimate relationship with the flow of qi. You might recall from Chapter 9 how the manifestation method of Huna, the Ha Ritual, is initiated by a breathing technique intended to build up the supply of *mana*—the Hawaiian word for qi or etheric energy.

Breathing patterns are also important in the practice of the martial arts. While these fighting arts certainly require a lot of training that is physical in nature, a true practitioner knows that their ultimate power derives from the invisible energy of the Etheric Body. That is why a kick or punch is made much more powerful by expelling a kiai—a short shout. Notice the word "ki" within "kiai." It is the etheric energy, *ki*, that enables a tiny and seemingly frail martial arts master to vanquish a much larger and physically stronger foe. This may be the stuff of legend and martial arts movies, but the etheric energy emanating from such masters has been measured and is real.[10]

Sound Therapies

In the etheric and higher energy realms, it's really all about vibration. Since physicists acknowledge that the subatomic components that ultimately make up our material world are likely vibrating strings of energy, conventional medicine uses vibrations of various kinds to heal too. Consider *histotripsy*, which uses targeted ultrasound to kill cancer cells. Radiation treatment could also be considered an etheric technique, despite its toxicity. In my view, both histotripsy and radiation treatment should be viewed as invasive.

From the physical to the etheric and beyond, it's all about vibes. So it's no surprise that ordinary sounds can have therapeutic power too. After all, sound is a vibration of air particles that reaches our eardrums and the hairs of our inner ears. Each of us who can hear or feel vibrations in our body knows that music and vibration can have a profound effect on our sense of well being. The fact that sound can affect us at every level, from physical to emotional, mental, and spiritual, has been used by every culture on Earth.

For instance, when we listen to particular kinds of music, we tend to feel more relaxed, happier, sadder, or more agitated. In India, certain *ragas* (traditional Indian musical motifs) are associated with specific moods and healing properties. And then, of course, we have shamans, who have always used chanting, drums, and rattles to create healing trance states. Meditators also utilize the power of sound when a gong or bell is utilized to open or close a meditative period. The horns, pipes, and drums of military forces have invoked bravery and power for thousands of years. In Jewish tradition, the blowing of the shofar, a ram's horn, creates an evocative herald of the New Year. Pacific Islanders blow the conch shell to mark the sunrise and sunset. All of these practices have profound effects because of the power of sound. Even animals are deeply affected by music and sound. Just search online for "animals affected by music." Sound truly has power.

Today, sound healing is beginning to emerge as a medicine of the 21ˢᵗ century. It all began during the 1930s with the modern ability to measure human brainwaves in certain states of consciousness (for example, alpha, beta, theta, and delta waves). In the 1950s and 1960s, the development of sound electronics and headphone technology enabled specific sounds to be directed into the ears in precise ways.

The most famous sound technology of this kind was developed by inventor and sound pioneer Robert Monroe, founder of the Monroe Institute.[11] In the early 1970s, he created the HemiSync, an audio technology that enables the brain to experience *binaural beats*—a phenomenon in which slightly different frequencies are delivered to each ear but are heard by the brain as a single tone. He soon discovered that this experience was associated with changes in consciousness, much like those experienced during meditation. Sometimes it even caused out-of-body experiences. Over time, Monroe and his growing group of followers found that the HemiSync can be tuned to enable *specific* altered states of consciousness. For example, through experimentation, they discovered how to use binaural beats to create desired emotional effects, like the reduction of anxiety or increased focus. They hypothesize that this occurs because the brain (and nervous system in general) tends to *synchronize* or resonate with these sounds. But perhaps it's the Etheric Body that is truly affected. Once again, it's about achieving similarity in vibration—the phenomenon that underlies the healing power of homeopathy. In fact, some homeopaths are now beginning to experiment with delivering remedies through sound.

Or consider Dr. Masuro Emoto's work with ice crystals. He played various sounds into water and then froze it. By doing so, he demonstrated, in a highly visual and dramatic way, that certain sounds, types of music, and even verbally expressed emotions, can create beauty or ugliness in physical form.[12]

Other types of sound healing have also been gaining popularity. One is the use of a traditional tool called a *singing bowl*—a metal or crystal bowl that can be struck or stroked in order to create a variety of sounds that have deep and penetrating emotional and healing effects. I once experienced this phenomenon at a singing bowl concert. I expected a performance of some kind, but instead, found that the experience caused emotional and physical effects in my body that lasted for a few days. Another fascinating body of work is described by sound therapist Eileen Day McKusick in her books *Tuning the Human Biofield* and *Electric Body, Electric Health*.[13] In them, she describes how her work with tuning forks has enabled her to not only discern patterns within the Etheric Body, but to effect cures in her clientele.

Certification programs are now being developed for the emerging practice of sound therapy. Such practitioners use tools like singing bowls, binaural beats, tuning forks, and mantras to deliver healing vibrations to their clients, and they are finding that specific locations within the physical and energetic bodies resonate with different sounds and tones. Sometimes sounds are even directed to specific points on the body, like the acupuncture points or chakras. I am certain that this form of healing will only grow in popularity over the next few decades.

Healing with Crystals and Geometry

I have now discussed how the Etheric Body is profoundly affected by vibration, whether it be encoded in sound or captured in the structured water of homeopathic remedies. Everything in nature manifests its own unique vibration—including you! Remarkably, it is also true of inanimate objects. Every culture on Earth has recognized this fact in its use of crystals, gems, and certain rocks for healing. These physical objects may hold the oldest forms of vibration on Earth and many people view them as possessing consciousness and wisdom too.

For instance, many minerals, and especially gems, have long been utilized to impart specific emotions and physical abilities, to energize, align and clear the physical and energy bodies, and to heal specific health problems. That is why shamans and monarchs have always worn gemstones or have utilized them in some other way. Some of their power may also arise from the *colors* they emanate—the visible vibrations of light.

Rocks and crystals can also be used to protect us from energies or to absorb them. Most people are aware of healing mineral baths—water impregnated not only with the minerals themselves, but with their energies too. And we all know that magnets can attract or repel energy. So it should be no surprise that certain nonmagnetic rocks can too. For example, a black carbon-based mineral found in Russia called *shungite* is now used for healing because it has been scientifically measured and proven in its ability to absorb EMFs.[14] In fact, I keep a shungite stone near my bed.

Of course, modern science also utilizes the vibratory nature of crystals for its own purposes. That's why quartz crystals are used to keep time in your watch and in computers. Many pharmaceutical drugs also include ground up minerals, though their developers likely do not understand the full energetic scope of their power.

How are minerals used for etheric healing in practice? Besides soaking in mineral baths, minerals are sometimes worn—on a necklace, ring, or in your pocket. Some practitioners place them on specific parts of your body, like the chakras, acupuncture points, or on locations where pain is occurring. Healing stones are also utilized to enhance focus and meditation. Some people arrange them into certain patterns in order to enhance their power as they communicate and trade energies with one another. Why not experiment with placing healing stones in certain locations around your home—for example, near your bed or in your car?

Incredibly, even structures and shapes can be used for healing too. This is the realm of *geometric healing*—the practice of utilizing objects with certain shapes or configurations to balance, enhance, or clear energy. Sitting inside pyramidal structures is one example. Another is the art of *Feng Shui*—an ancient Chinese form of geometric knowledge that has gained much popularity in recent years as an interior design technique.[15] Feng Shui recognizes that the placement of doors, windows, mirrors, lights, and furniture within a room dramatically affects the energy and thus the experience of the people who dwell within it. Feng Shui principles also recognize the importance of alignment with respect to the magnetic field of the Earth—north, south, east, and west.

Finally, consider the work of Egyptian scientist and architect Dr. Ibrahim Karim, who spent 40 years developing a science he calls *Biogeometry*.[16] Perhaps it is only fitting that this system emerges from Egypt, given its historical association with pyramids. Dr. Karim's work is based on the idea that certain geometric forms impart specific *qualities* of energy. In particular, he identified a centering energy existing within all living systems that he called BG3, which can be detected and measured in terms of three energy qualities. Karim then developed specific shapes that interact with the Etheric Body to amplify BG3 and harmonize bodily energy interactions with the environment. These shapes can be embedded in medallions that are worn or constructed as three-dimensional objects.

Being a scientist, Dr. Karim has performed extensive research with these shapes. For example, he conducted successful medical experiments focused on healing farm animals. A larger scale experiment was undertaken by the Swiss town of Hemberg to alleviate the suffering of residents who became ill due to various forms of EMFs and geopathic stress (energies emanating from the Earth itself). Another town in Switzerland called Hirschberg also implemented Karim's biogeometric solutions and found that they not only helped with electromagnetic sensitivity but also had positive effects on the ecology of the region. Amazing! Given that EMFs are likely to become even more pervasive, Dr. Karim's benign geometric solutions may become extremely important for all of us.

Muscle Testing (Applied Kinesiology)

Another technique that many alternative therapists utilize is muscle testing, sometimes called applied kinesiology. Although it is not a therapy in itself, muscle testing is used by practitioners to determine whether a particular therapeutic choice will be useful to a patient. The idea is that the strength of a specific muscle, usually an arm muscle, is affected by responses to a treatment within the Etheric Body, and then, by extension the Physical Body.

In essence, muscle testing is a kind of biofeedback tool. The therapist "applies" a particular therapeutic choice—for example, having a patient hold a specific remedy or supplement, or asking the patient a question—and then seeing how that choice affects muscle strength. I've included this technique in this chapter because it is the response of the Etheric Body that is considered to affect the tested muscle. However, the technique supposedly also works if the muscle of a surrogate is used instead—even at a distance. If this is true, it indicates that muscle testing can operate via the Astral Body as well.

Which brings us now to consider the Astral, Mental, and Causal Bodies—the bodies that we take with us after we die and our Etheric Body dissipates. In the next three chapters, I will discuss how healing these enduring parts of your complete Self can have even more powerful effects.

CHAPTER 16

WE ARE EMOTIONAL
PSYCHIC BEINGS

Most of us struggle at times with a health problem. Usually, we try all kinds of physical interventions to alleviate it, and when these fail, we may utilize something more esoteric like homeopathy or acupuncture. But what if these fail too? What to do? That's when it's time to dig deeper.

I already told you about my own struggle with insomnia. Naturally, I tried the usual physical interventions—removing the TV from the bedroom, eliminating all room lights after bedtime, limiting nighttime exposure to blue light, avoiding drinking liquids late in the evening in order to reduce nighttime urination, taking magnesium to relax my body, listening to soothing sounds, and more. These measures did help, but they didn't solve my problem. I also tried homeopathy, my go-to medicine, but it didn't help that much either. Eventually, I realized that it was time to penetrate even deeper into the core of my being—the part of me that exists beyond my physical or even my Etheric Body: my Astral Body.

As I discussed in Part II, the higher energy bodies—the Astral, Mental, and Causal Bodies—continue to exist even after our Physical Body crumbles to dust and its etheric energy dissipates. For almost all of us, these higher bodies will eventually be reincarnated for another go round, another stab at learning and evolving on the physical plane. But even while we are in physical form, these energetic parts of us are still able to express themselves in very physical ways. They are also important subjects of study by many disciplines, though they may go by different names.

The Astral Body, the emotional and psychic seat of our being, is often called the subconscious or unconscious mind, though its scope and powers go way beyond what psychology ascribes to it. For example, there are aspects of the Astral Body that are quite conscious to us; you are certainly aware of many of your emotions. Your Astral Body also stores all of your memories. (No, they are not simply stored in your brain, although the brain does perform work in service to the Astral Body.) And it is the astral part of you that enables you to have psychic perceptions. It also plays a critical role in your physical and emotional health.

One of the reasons why astral issues are so impactful is that our Astral and Etheric Bodies are highly interwoven and communicate with one another constantly. That's why our feelings, whether they be conscious or unconscious, quickly affect us in very physical ways. For example, your emotional feelings trigger the release of chemicals that affect your organs and bodily systems. Even allopathic doctors acknowledge this. Indeed, the awareness that emotional stress is one of the leading causes of disease has become downright mainstream. But what doctors usually don't fully understand is *how* all of this happens. It's not simply about neurochemicals and hormones. Instead, the unseen Astral Body communicates its energetic feelings to the Etheric Body, which then, in turn, transmits that information to the Physical Body. Thus, stress hormones are only the *end product* of emotions in the Astral Body and not the *root* cause of ill health.

Because the Astral Body plays such a key role in our health and well-being, it is the focus of a great number of healing modalities that have become increasingly popular today. In indigenous cultures, however, the role of the Astral Body has long been acknowledged. Yes, shamans may utilize herbal medicines and various etheric tools as part of their repertoire, but the astral level is probably the most important arena in which they work. For instance, a skilled shaman often operates by cajoling the Astral Body towards health, removing harmful astral influences or attachments, and even working with groups of astral bodies within family units or communities.

For all of these reasons, finding an astral-level healing tool that works for you is probably one of the most important things you can do to attain physical and emotional health and change your life for the better. I know it's been true for me. In fact, healing at this level is probably the answer for *most* of our so-called "physical" problems, including musculoskeletal pain, high blood pressure, chronic eczema, migraines, and more. Don't forget, the deeper the level a healing tool is working at, the broader its potential scope of power. So even if you can't afford a doctor, homeopath, acupuncturist, or herbalist, you can still work with your Astral Body on your own.

SIGNS AND CAUTIONS FOR THE ASTRAL REALM

Before we get into detail about the basic principles and healing tools that operate at the astral level, let's begin with some signs that a problem is rooted in this realm, along with some cautionary advice.

Signs that your problem may be astrally-based

First, remember that although your problem may be manifesting as physical symptoms like severe pain, and even if you have medical evidence of physical malfunction, your issue may still be rooted and healed in a non-physical way. Don't forget: your mind and emotions ultimately control your body via their interactions with the Etheric Body. Do not believe otherwise! In fact, your rational thinking mind will probably try to convince you *not* to engage with astral level healing because it doesn't want you to dig deeper and discover what's *truly* going on "under the hood" of conscious awareness.

Dr. John Sarno, a pioneer in astral-level healing (although he would likely have balked at the word "astral"), identified a certain class of people who are especially prone to manifesting emotional problems in a physical way. He called them "goodists." These are folks who tend to suppress their anger, or at least try to always be nice, helpful, and kind. In fact, goodists would rather turn their anger inward and blame themselves than outwardly express it in some way. As a result, their negative feelings are often buried and suppressed and become completely unconscious to them. Most women are acculturated by society to operate in this way, which is why they tend to fall into this category more often than men. Still, many men are goodists too. Goodists also tend to have difficulty saying "no." They want to be liked and responsible, and are often hard-working students and achievers. Society loves and rewards its goodists, which is another reason why so many of us suffer from physical problems that are actually rooted at the astral level.

Do you doubt that your conscious or subconscious emotional state could be causing physical symptoms? Consider the following list of complaints that Dr. Sarno successfully treated in a non-physical way:

- Musculoskeletal pain almost anywhere in the body, but especially in the back, neck, and joints, as well as problems with tendons

- Spinal or peripheral nerve tingling or other nerve-related symptoms

- Gastroesophageal reflux (GERD) and spasm

- Ulcers

- Hiatal hernia

- Irritable bowel syndrome (IBS)

- Spastic colitis

- Tension or migraine headache

- Frequent urination, especially at night

- Prostatitis

- Sexual dysfunction

- Tinnitus

- Dizziness

Sarno believed that the Astral Body (which he called the unconscious or subconscious mind) tends to express itself as a specific physical problem that it believes you will "buy into." For example, it often creates a "disease du-jour." Forty years ago the problem would likely have been a stomach ulcer. Twenty years ago it was probably lower back pain. Later it became carpal tunnel syndrome. Today it might be wandering chronic pain or insomnia. The media certainly provide a plethora of additional "nocebos"—negative health messages—that your Astral Body can also latch onto and utilize as part of its repertoire.

Here are some more clues that your problems might be astral in nature:

- The problems began after an emotional upset or trauma. Be aware that you may have completely forgotten about this trigger. It may even be something seemingly benign, like an upsetting TV show or conversation.

- You have not been helped or have only been palliated by physical and etheric healing strategies.

- Symptoms are out of proportion to the injury or event that supposedly precipitated them, or have never been triggered by similar events in the past.

- Symptoms come and go, or move around from place to place.

- Your symptoms have a symbolic analogue. For example, if you have urinary issues, you may actually be "pissed" at someone or about something. Or you may be arguing with someone who is literally "a pain in the neck" or you can't "stomach" something you have to deal with.

- You have a history of physical or emotional childhood abuse, abandonment, or neglect.

- You have a tendency toward addictions of various kinds, including the modern varieties: shopping, eating, sex, social media, news watching, gaming, and other distracting entertainment.

- You have been subjected to a toxic work or relationship environment.

- You tend to suppress or not be in touch with your feelings. This may also be a familial tendency or pattern.

Signs that a problem is not just astral and might be better helped by approaches at the mental or causal levels

If all therapies at the physical, etheric, and astral levels have not helped, consider mental level therapies. One key characteristic of Mental Body problems is that they pertain to life meaning—for example, if you are struggling to understand your purpose in life. Signs of Causal Body dysfunction include feeling disconnected from spirit and not knowing who you are. These deeper problems also tend to express themselves in significant dreams, though dysfunctions at all levels can be communicated in this way too.

Cautions for astral level treatment

It is very important to realize that working at the astral level may be emotionally painful. This is because many of the feelings of the Astral Body are subconscious (especially the ones that manifest in physical problems), and are subconscious for a reason: some part of you does not want to face them. As a result, discovering and releasing these memories and feelings will be resisted. However, if you keep at it and *do* push through, the results can be unbelievably liberating. In fact, you may end up changing your entire life for the better.

Many astral-level healing methods can be attempted on your own, especially with the aid of books or online teachings. Still, you might need to seek out a practitioner. Remember that practitioner certification is always preferable and that recommendations can be helpful. Also trust your intuitions and sensations when working with any practitioner. If you suspect that a therapy or practitioner is not for you, discontinue treatment. Because astral-level problems are often chronic in nature, you will likely be visiting a practitioner regularly, at least for a while. Because they will be delving into a deep and emotional aspect of your being, it is important that your relationship with them be comfortable and trusting.

ASTRAL BODY RECAP

Before I get into more detail about astral level healing, it may be useful to review the nature of this realm. Our Astral Body is a distinct and extremely powerful part of us that continues on after our death. Indeed, one of the main reasons we reincarnate is to further develop and evolve this part of us. Esoteric teacher and visionary, G.I. Gurdjieff,[1] believed that, eventually, our Astral Body evolves to become a Mental Body and no longer needs to incarnate into physical form. Later, it may then evolve into a purely causal being, merged into oneness with God and creation. But the truth is, almost all of us have *many* more cycles of reincarnation and evolution to complete before we reach that point!

Here, once again, are some of the main characteristics of the Astral Body:

- It is our most important conduit between our higher energy bodies and our Etheric Body, and thus plays a vital role in our physical health.

- It stores all of our memories and beliefs (conscious and unconscious).

- It is the primary source of our inner emotions and feelings.

- It has no rational or reasoning ability (the domain of the Mental Body).

- It is the primary source of our psychic abilities and connections.

- It is highly impressed and affected by our physical senses, including hearing, sight, smell, and touch.

- It is generally obedient and subservient to the Mental and Causal Bodies.

Boiling all of this down: *when it comes to the Astral Body, it's all about feelings and beliefs.* And these feelings and beliefs are powerful! They can create disease and they can heal us; they can age us or they can rejuvenate us. And there's lots of scientific evidence for this. One of the most fascinating books on this topic is *Counterclockwise* by psychologist Ellen Langer.[2] In it, she describes several studies that prove that belief and feelings *do* create our physical reality.

Probably the most famous of Langer's experiments was conducted in 1979 on a group of men in their late seventies and early eighties. The test subjects were measured before and after the experiment for things like dexterity, flexibility, vision, sensitivity to taste, visual memory, intellectual abilities like completing mazes, physical appearance, and psychological state of mind. The experimental group spent a week at a retreat center that was carefully designed to look and feel like the year 1959. In fact, the men were instructed to pretend that they were actually 20 years younger. They were not allowed to discuss anything that happened after 1959 and were instructed to talk in the present tense, as if it were truly September 1959. Discussion groups focused on current events of the time, TV shows and movies, and more. In contrast, the control group also spent time at the same retreat center, but was not told to pretend they were living in 1959. As a result, theirs was simply a nostalgic experience, reminiscing about their lives 20 years before.

What were the results? Both groups changed in behavior and attitude as a result of the experiment. They became more self-sufficient, and their hearing, memory, and grip strength improved. However, the experimental group showed greater improvement in joint flexibility as well as in height, gait, and posture, diminishment of arthritis, and higher scores on the intelligence tests. Objective observers who were given photos of the men taken before and after the experiment judged the experimental group to be much younger in appearance. You do indeed become what you believe!

Just think about the implications of this experiment. Consider the fact that societal messages about old age may actually be *making them so*, and that we could improve health outcomes significantly for our elders by simply treating them as if they were young and healthy instead of infirm.

What we believe about our daily activities can also change how they affect us, as was shown in another experiment described in *Counterclockwise*. An experimental group of hotel cleaners were told that their daily room-cleaning activities were excellent forms of exercise, whereas the control group did not receive this message. Amazingly, the cleaners who believed they were exercising at work experienced weight loss, increased muscle mass, and other benefits of exercise. The control group did not, even though they performed the same activities. Other studies have shown that simply imagining or visualizing that you are doing strenuous exercise builds muscle too!

The bottom line is that our memories, beliefs, and emotions do affect our Physical Body in remarkable ways. But remember: the Astral Body is also impressionable and subservient in nature and has no rational or logical ability of its own. It believes what it hears or sees. Thus, if you watch a horror movie, your Astral Body believes that the horrors have actually occurred and will create physiological changes in response. And if someone—especially an authority figure you trust—tells you something about your health, your Astral Body will try to make it so. That's why placebos and, perhaps more importantly, *nocebos* can affect us so profoundly.

Most of us have heard the term "placebo" and know that it's usually used in a derogatory way. But the fact is, the power of the placebo effect is awesome and used by doctors every day. If a health practitioner tells you that a pill or treatment will cure you, your Astral Body will hear, believe, and make it so. Experiments have even shown that performing sham knee surgeries can have the same result as doing the real thing. So if you can be cured by a harmless pill or treatment, isn't that preferable to taking a toxic drug or undergoing surgery? Of course! (However, lest you believe that therapies like homeopathy are working by placebo alone, know that the whole concept of a placebo-controlled test was designed by homeopaths in the 1800s in order to prove that the efficacy of homeopathic remedies goes beyond the placebo effect. In fact, many recent studies have also shown this to be the case.)

But what about a *nocebo*? It's a negative health message, and you will find them swarming around you every day. Every advertisement for a pharmaceutical drug, every alert about an epidemic disease and the need to be vaccinated, every dire health warning and directive to be screened for every possible disease—these can act as nocebos. Indeed, when a doctor pronounces that a patient only has "three months to live," the patient's Astral Body will sometimes hear and comply, causing the patient to die on the prescribed date.

Truly, the dire pronouncements made by doctors or other authorities may be no different than those of sorcerers who throw curses upon their victims. For example, Joe Dispenza's book *You Are the Placebo*[3] includes an anecdote about an advanced cancer patient who was told that a new alternative treatment would cure him. When he received the treatment, the cancer disappeared. A few months later, however, the man read an article stating that the treatment he had received was a sham. His cancer quickly returned and he died.

So why are we constructed this way? Why give such immense power to our suggestible Astral Body? Perhaps because it's a very effective way for us to get useful feedback. If our beliefs can create our reality, then our experienced reality tells us something about our beliefs. For example, if you are always experiencing misfortunes, you may conclude that you are a hapless victim of circumstance. But think again! Maybe it is your *belief* in your victimhood that has trapped you. Luckily, you can then change your beliefs and emotions to be more positive and have more positive outcomes. As Joe Dispenza says, "Your personality creates your personal-reality."

Also, don't forget that the Astral Body is highly impressed by physical senses and actions. So just *thinking* more positive beliefs may not be enough. You need to *do* something. You might work with an astral healer, perform a ritual or ceremony, listen to healing information on a hypnosis tape, recite affirmations, or simply write down your inner feelings and say them out loud. When you do, your Astral Body will notice and listen. And that's what astral level healing is all about—getting in sync with your emotional inner being, listening to it with compassion, and helping it to grow and evolve.

ASTRALLY-BASED THERAPIES

Now let's consider some astral-level therapies in more detail. Below is a list of the ones I'll cover in this chapter, though there are many more out there. Also know that some of these modalities operate at the mental and causal levels too.

Approaches that work by simply acknowledging the powerful role of the Astral Body

- The work of Dr. John Sarno and TMS

Communicate with your Astral Body

- Psychotherapy

- Hypnotherapy

- Journaling, Meditation, Divination

- Mirror Work, Self-compassion, Self-love

- The Sedona Method

- Core Transformation

- Family Constellation Therapy

Connect with the Astral Body via the Physical Body

- EFT (Emotional Freedom Technique) and TFT (Thought Field Therapy)

- EMDR (Eye Movement Desensitization and Reprocessing)

- TRE (Trauma Release Exercises)

- Breathwork, Sweat Lodges, Ecstatic Dance, Sound, and Plant Medicine

- Shamanism

SIMPLY ACKNOWLEDGE THE POWERFUL ROLE OF THE ASTRAL BODY

The work of Dr. John Sarno and TMS

Long before I knew anything about homeopathy or had any real interest in alternative medicine, I often suffered from lower back pain. It all began when I was fifteen, soon after my father died, but I didn't really try to do anything about it until I was in graduate school. I have a clear memory of going to my first chiropractor at that time and getting some good results. After that experience, I religiously performed the exercises he recommended whenever my back acted up.

A few years later, however, exercise and chiropractic were not doing the trick. That's when someone suggested that I read a new book that was getting quite the buzz—*Mind Over Back Pain* by Dr. John Sarno, MD.[4] I still remember lying in bed immobilized by pain and reading Sarno's short 128-page treatise. In it, he explained his theory about *Tension Myositis Syndrome* or *TMS*. Sarno claimed that his patients only needed to accept that their pain was emotional in origin in order to achieve a cure. After some introspection, I followed his advice, and within a day or two I was pain free! In fact, I've never had as much of a problem with lower back pain since that time. When I do, the first thing I do is try to figure out what is bothering me emotionally.

How could reading a book and believing what it said free me from years of occasional lower back pain? Well, it was about accepting the true origin of my pain: suppressed negative emotions. In other words, by simply believing that my back pain was not due to any physical defect and by acknowledging that it was my own subconscious feelings and thoughts that created it, my pain disappeared. In fact, these days, whenever I experience that familiar back twinge, I usually don't need to delve any deeper than that. Nor do I need to dredge up old memories from the past or see a therapist. I just need to believe and acknowledge that my back pain has originated in what I now call my Astral Body.

Of course, Dr. Sarno never used the term "Astral Body." He was a confirmed allopath and a professor of rehabilitative medicine at the NYU medical school. He had plenty of experience treating back and other musculoskeletal pain. But as he described in *Mind Over Back Pain*, over the years, he had begun to notice that his patients tended to share certain psychological traits—what he called "goodist" qualities, which I described earlier in this chapter. Sarno also came to realize that standard allopathic treatments often only worked for a short period of time, after which a patient's problems returned. Indeed, this was true even after surgery. He also observed that pain symptoms were sometimes inconsistent with diagnosed physical pathology, and that the pains could inexplicably wander from place to place. In medical journals, he even read about people with verifiable "slipped disc" or other physiological abnormalities who didn't experience pain at all. How could that be?

Dr. Sarno did acknowledge that his patients' pain was real and not due to hysteria or some kind of ploy to get attention; it wasn't "all in their heads." He became determined to find some physiological explanation for it. Ultimately he came up with the answer: the syndrome he called TMS. Its mechanism is surprisingly simple too. Rather than arising from a physical defect like nerve compression (even if the defect is verified by imaging or some other test), TMS pain is caused by *muscular tension*. Indeed, this tension might be very subtle and go unnoticed by both patient and doctor. Nevertheless, it can still cause a reduction in blood flow to the tissues, with the net effect being depleted oxygen supply and the resulting pain. Simple!

So, what's causing this muscular tension? It's not very hard to figure out. We all know that stress and other negative emotions can cause our muscles to tense up. It's built into our "fight, flight, freeze" response. But when we don't really need to fight or run away, and even when we don't consciously realize that we're angry or afraid, our muscles *still* tense up. Even if this tension is subtle and largely unconscious, if it's also persistent, it can result in TMS and pain.

Sarno's treatment regimen was quite simple and he had amazing curative success, even in cases with verifiable physiological pathology and repeated unsuccessful surgeries. The first and critical step was to explain the TMS theory to the patient and convince them to accept a TMS diagnosis. Interestingly, certain characteristics of TMS are also indicative of issues originating in the Astral Body: pain that moves from location to location over time (something very common today among people with a "chronic pain" diagnosis); pain that is out of proportion to the supposed injury that triggered it, or is attributed to something that never caused a problem before; a "goodist" personality (described in the Signs and Cautions section); and a history of childhood abuse, neglect, or some other psychological trauma. Once a TMS diagnosis is understood and accepted by a patient, they are instructed to go about their daily activities (including sports), even when they experience pain. Amazingly, a good proportion of patients completely recover within a period of weeks after this step alone.

For some people, however, it's not that easy. For them, a big obstacle is getting them to truly accept the diagnosis. Remember that the cause of TMS is *suppressed* emotions, and for many people, these emotions have been suppressed for a reason. Maybe they are simply too painful to feel or are associated with memories that are too traumatic to remember. According to Sarno, the most common emotions suppressed in TMS are anger and rage, and the most common reason for suppressing them is that they are viewed as *unacceptable.*

Basically, it boils down to the Astral Body trying to be obedient—to be "good." It believes that producing physical pain is preferable to dredging up and expressing anger or rage or some other form of emotional pain. In essence, pain serves as an ideal distraction mechanism—because if you are in pain, it's hard to think about anything else! Moreover, the Astral Body believes that lying in bed with a "slipped disc" or missing work because of "carpal tunnel syndrome" is much more socially acceptable than letting out a tirade of anger and rage.

But even if a TMS diagnosis is accepted, Sarno found that some people need more help. His first approach was to have them join a support group. He also suggested that patients write down and say out loud everything that is bothering them. Personally, I have found this journaling method to be particularly helpful. But if these steps are still not enough, Sarno recommended counseling.

One thing that many TMS patients experience is that, after their original pain disappears, something new crops up. Sarno called this phenomenon the "symptom imperative." For example, instead of back pain, a patient may now suffer from neck or elbow pain or perhaps gastrointestinal problems. Sarno's theory was that once the subconscious mind realizes that the original physical problem is no longer working as an effective distraction, it decides to try some new ache or pain. Remember, if a patient is prone to TMS, they are likely to remain so. That's why Sarno always educated his patients to remain vigilant and reapply TMS awareness whenever new problems crop up.

Dr. Sarno's amazing successes with TMS treatment eventually made him a controversial figure within the medical community. When he expanded his theory to explain (and heal) not only musculoskeletal pain but almost every type of illness (see his final book, *The Divided Mind*), he became even more of a pariah. It's easy to see why. If pain and disease can be treated by simply acknowledging the role of the subconscious mind, how would doctors make a living and the pharmaceutical companies reap their profits?

If you're interested in learning more about TMS, I suggest reading one of Dr. Sarno's books. Then put the ideas into practice. The next time you get a pain in your back or neck or even come down with a cold, stomachache, or headache, take a good look within and ask yourself: Am I angry about something? Am I afraid of something? Sometimes this step alone is enough and the problem will pass.

If not, buy a journal and write down everything, big or small, that is bothering you. I have a journal for this purpose. For each entry, I write the date and the words "What's bugging me?" Then I let it all out. No one but you should read this journal. The process is even more effective if you privately read what you have written out loud. Remember that physical actions (like writing and speaking) impress your Astral Body and let it know you are listening. If Sarno was correct and TMS is a distraction mechanism, you are essentially telling the Astral Body that you'd rather feel your emotions than be in physical distress.

Actually, my own theory for why TMS occurs is a bit different from Sarno's, though the net effect is the same. Rather than trying to distract you, I believe that the goal of the Astral Body is to *communicate* with you. When you write your angst down and read it out loud, you are telling it that you are listening and its message has been received. If you also meditate and try to connect with your Astral Body more deeply, your healing can be even more effective.

One last interesting note about Dr. Sarno. If you read his books, you will discover that he was not a fan of alternative medicine. He believed that all treatment methods besides allopathy operate strictly via the placebo effect. The difference between Sarno and the skeptics, however, is that he acknowledged that his own methods operated in the same way and that the "placebo effect" is essentially the amazing power of the subconscious mind (part of the Astral Body) to create both disease *and* healing.

COMMUNICATE WITH YOUR ASTRAL BODY

Psychotherapy

Naturally, sometimes simply acknowledging the role of your Astral Body isn't enough. You need to dive deeper, make contact with this part of your greater Self, and have a real conversation. The most traditional way to do this is to work with a psychotherapist. When doctors like Sigmund Freud and Carl Jung first developed and expanded the field of psychiatry in the 1800s and 1900s, their goal was to access the memories and feelings of the subconscious minds of their patients. Carl Jung then went beyond Freud in recognizing the importance of *synchronicity* (in fact, he coined the term) as a way to communicate with and understand the astral realm.

Unfortunately, after the 1960s, psychiatry shifted its focus to the use of pharmaceutical drugs. As a result, working with a psychologist or a non-medical counseling professional is now the only way people usually try to make contact with their Astral Body. The number of approaches utilized by such therapists is vast and beyond the scope of this book. Most techniques help patients to uncover their family history and understand how it affects their emotional patterns and coping strategies. These practitioners also try to help patients navigate their lives and relationships more skillfully. This can be extremely helpful, but in some ways, it provides information that is more useful to the rational Mental Body than to the emotional Astral Body. The bottom line is that, in order to truly heal at the astral level, you must make earnest contact with this part of yourself and not simply intellectually understand it better. If you do, it can provide great relief to your Astral Body, which tends to be subservient to the Mental Body and often feels unheard.

So how *does* your Astral Body—your powerful yet often childlike inner being—actually feel? What does it *really* want? Most importantly, how can you help it to release (not suppress) its sometimes destructive emotional patterns and move into a healthier and happier state of being? The rest of this chapter will describe many tools for doing so, including working with a psychotherapist.

Over the years, psychologists have come up with a variety of ways to contact the Astral Body. Among them are dream interpretation, hypnosis, word association, various forms of artistic expression, meditation, and more. I have personally benefited by working with therapists using such techniques. Some have even helped me to recover a few past life memories. This can be extremely helpful because, whether we consciously remember them or not, past lives continue to exist within the astral realm and can affect our Astral Body in this life.

Some people, however, have no problem letting their Astral Body express itself. These people have a very dominating (rather than subservient) Astral Body and often behave like toddlers having a temper tantrum. In other words, they don't allow their rational Mental Body to limit them very much. Despite their acting out, however, such folks still have buried astral feelings. Narcissists, for example, typically have very low self-esteem that is unconscious to them. Unfortunately, psychotherapy can be challenging for such individuals. Successful treatment tends to focus on increasing *rational* awareness of their problematic behavior and providing them with tools to foster behavioral change. In other words, therapy for narcissists is more about getting their Astral Body to align with the rational directives of their Mental Body.

Finally, if you do decide to work with a psychotherapist, know that the therapeutic process usually consists of weekly sessions that may go on for months or even years. Group therapy is also an option. Because of this, it is important that you trust and click with your therapist or group and feel comfortable with them.

Hypnotherapy

When most of us think of hypnotism, we imagine a stage show with a hypnotist who puts an unwitting victim under a trance and tells them to do embarrassing things—perhaps, barking like a dog or prancing about like a chicken. Then, when the hypnotized subject is brought out of the trance state, they have no memory of what occurred. While this stereotype of hypnotism may have a grain of truth to it, rest assured that going to a hypnotherapist is nothing like that! In fact, very few people have the level of suggestibility depicted in such stage acts.

The underlying idea behind hypnotherapy is very much in line with everything I have written about the Astral and Mental Bodies. In particular, it acknowledges that the Astral Body is: (1) generally subservient to the rational Mental Body; (2) highly impressed by what it sees and hears; and (3) able to control physical changes and behaviors, even without the cooperation or acknowledgement of the Mental Body.

Given these assumptions, the goal of the hypnotherapist is to first, subdue the limiting power of the rational Mental Body so that the Astral Body can be reached without interference from inhibiting thoughts. This step, called *induction*, is achieved through a variety of simple techniques that turn down the volume of the rational thinking mind. Certain eye movements, breathing patterns, a darkened room, lying down, etc. can achieve it. Essentially, the hypnotherapist places the patient in a kind of twilight or trance state, similar to the point between waking consciousness and sleep. In modern brain-wave terminology, the patient's brain waves are coaxed from the waking beta-wave state into a predominantly alpha-wave or even theta-wave or delta-wave state—a state of relaxed wakefulness.

Once this has been achieved, the Astral Body can be reached and influenced more easily. The hypnotherapist then gives the Astral Body specific suggestions, based on the needs of the patient. For example, a hypnotic suggestion might be to release a phobia or fear, achieve weight loss, stop smoking, or have a more healthy relationship. When the suggestion is complete, the hypnotherapist slowly guides the patient back into normal waking consciousness.

I first visited a hypnotherapist to help me with my chronic insomnia. While it did not cure the problem, after two or three sessions with the therapist, it definitely eased my anxiety around sleep. I never became unconscious of what was going on during these sessions; perhaps I am not easily put into a trance, which may also explain my only moderate success. Still, I found the whole experience extremely helpful.

The beginning of a hypnotherapy session is much like a visit to a psychotherapist. In my case, I discussed my problem for about 30 minutes, including my psychological insights into its origin. The rest of the appointment lasted about 15-20 minutes. First, the room was darkened. Next, I laid back in a recliner and the therapist guided me through some simple exercises to relax and enter a very light trance. She then provided suggestions about releasing my anxieties and having successful, restful sleep. I found it particularly helpful when she told me that even if I wasn't sleeping, all was well and I was fine. I was then brought out of the trance state. A recording of the hypnosis segment of the session was also provided to me, which I could listen to any time, especially before bedtime.

If you are interested in this form of therapy, know that hypnotherapists charge at about the same rate as psychologists. However, rather than ongoing weekly sessions, only a few hypnotherapy sessions are typically suggested or required. For common issues, it may not even be necessary to see a hypnotherapist at all. You can buy hypnosis tapes for a variety of problems that you can use before sleep or at any other time—but not when you need to be awake or alert. My own hypnotherapist, Alba Alamillo, provides several free hypnosis videos on her YouTube channel, and she also wrote a useful and amusing book about hypnosis and the subconscious mind that I highly recommend.[5] Be aware that some hypnosis tapes mask the sound of the hypnotist's voice with natural sounds like ocean waves. These so-called *subliminal* tapes can work because the Astral Body can still receive suggestions, even if the conscious mind cannot.

Journaling, Meditation, Automatic Writing, and Divination Methods

You can also make contact and communicate with your Astral Body on your own. I've already discussed one method—journaling. I recommend having a special journal just for this purpose. When you feel the need, let it all hang out and write down everything that is bothering you, from big to small and even petty. Then be sure to read what you have written out loud.

You'll be surprised at how effective this simple procedure can be. In fact, it helped me recover from a severe case of sciatica. Several years ago, I began experiencing pain shooting down my left leg. Initially, it started as a mild ache. But as the weeks progressed, it got much worse. Since I was already familiar with Dr. Sarno's teachings, I tried to tell myself "it's just stress and will pass," but the pain continued to worsen, even after several trips to the osteopath. After about a month, I was using a cane to walk and had to sleep propped up in bed with my leg raised on pillows. Eventually, I needed to sleep in a recliner. On top of this, my husband and I had a trip planned to New Zealand and Australia just a few weeks later to visit our son. I needed to take action quickly!

I began by rereading Sarno's book, journaling each day, and reading out loud what I had written. I also spent time trying to remember what was going on at the time the pain began. In homeopathy, identifying the causative event for an illness can be important for finding the correct remedy, so I figured that this might be a critical step. After looking back through my personal diary, I discovered that at just about the time the pain began, I had an upsetting conversation with my son who lived in Sydney. Apparently, I had suppressed my emotional reaction and had even forgotten about the incident. I now recalled that it had actually been quite intense for me. No doubt the sciatica was doing its job as a distraction! Or perhaps, my Astral Body was trying to express itself in a physical way. In either case, remembering this conversation was a very important step in solving my sciatica pain.

Armed with this new information, I began to focus my journaling on my feelings about what had happened with my son. As I lay in my recliner (which by now had taken up residence in the bedroom), I let it all out in written form, followed by an impassioned oral reading session. Amazingly, within a day or so, the pain began to subside. I also had a heart-to-heart phone conversation with my son about the incident. A week later, I was completely pain free, felt better about my relationship with my son, and went on a wonderful trip. Success!

Another way to make contact with your Astral Body is to meditate. This works because quieting your busy mind makes room for astral emotions to arise and be felt. Although some people try to focus their meditation on contacting their wise Causal Body, making contact with your Astral Body can be just as important, especially when it comes to your health. When you do, remember that your Astral Body often has a childlike quality to it. You might even find it helpful to try to visualize what it looks like. Does your Astral Body seem to be male or female? How old is it? What is the expression on his or her face? How does it feel and what does it want you to know? What words of encouragement, understanding, and compassion can you give to this part of your Self?

Also remember that merely "thinking" to your Astral Body is usually not as effective as *doing* something. For example, you might try an interesting journaling technique called *automatic writing*. I sometimes use it if I get an intuitive feeling that some form of contact is trying to be made from one of my higher bodies. Begin by entering a light meditative state. Then, start your journal entry by addressing this part of yourself (for example, "Dear Astral Body"). Then, write down a question. It might be specific or as general as, "What do you want to tell me?" or "What is important for me to know?"

Now write an open quotation mark (") and let the words flow out of you. Try not to think about what you are writing or to write in a grammatical way; just let the words come out. As you do so, you may experience a sensation that feels like you are receiving information from some external source, not your own mind. Eventually, you will have another sensation that lets you know the message is complete. After a few minutes or later in the day, review what you have written. The results of this practice can often be quite surprising and profound.

Another way to make contact with your Astral Body is through one of many types of *divination*. Typical examples include the use of tarot or animal cards, throwing I-Ching coins, or dowsing with a crystal hanging by a thread. Divination works because you are receiving information through the mechanism of synchronicity. In other words, if you ask a question, the answer delivered to you as a card choice, coin toss, or pendulum swing synchronistically represents your answer. Since the astral realm is also the domain of psychic phenomena, it is easy for your Astral Body to communicate with you in this way.

Please note that if you'd like to use divination as a communication method, your success will improve over time if you keep using the same divination tool. In essence, you are training your Astral Body to open up and communicate with you in a particular way. When you use this tool repeatedly, it slowly becomes *conditioned* to you, and the more conditioned it becomes, the more accurate it is.

Another way to communicate with your Astral Body is to simply talk out loud to it. Imagine that it is a young person who simply needs love and encouragement. Sometimes your Astral Body becomes locked in a state you experienced during childhood, usually as a way to survive. If painful memories from the past arise during your conversation, tell this younger, inner part of you that everything is all right and that you love them. Give them a hug! You might imagine your current self as an angel that is helping your younger self, nurturing it lovingly as it experiences painful past scenarios.

Another helpful technique is to replay a past painful event in your mind while modifying it so that it has a positive outcome. This may sound dubious, but it can work and be quite healing. Who knows? Maybe a part of you *is* going back in time and assuaging that hurt little child or creating a new timeline where events turn out for the better. After all, the Astral Body is higher dimensional and can move through space and time at will.

Mirror Work, Self-compassion, Self-love

Another way to express compassion for your inner Astral Body is to engage in *mirror work*. Using a small hand mirror or some other mirror around your house, look deeply into your own eyes and tell yourself (out loud) how much you love yourself and how wonderful and beautiful you are. Try to do this every day, repeatedly, using a variety of words and affirmations.

This may sound rather simplistic and easy to perform, but believe me, it can be quite difficult—at least, initially. It is also a highly emotional practice that can transform not only your own life experience, but your relationships with others as well. How so? Because when you learn to love and accept yourself, you not only become happier and healthier within, but you are freed up to have more love and compassion for others.

Mirror work was most famously promulgated by Louise Hay,[6] an important teacher in the self-help movement and founder of Hay House Publishing. Both my husband Steve and I took one of her online mirror work courses and found it to be extremely helpful. Indeed, I think courses like this should be made a part of every elementary school curriculum. Our whole society would change for the better as a result.

Louise Hay's backstory is a fascinating one. After an extremely difficult childhood of abuse, she discovered the principles of the *Science of Mind*, most famously taught by New Thought leader Ernest Holmes.[7]

Put simply, the Science of Mind teaches that we each create a life that reflects what we believe and think. As a result, changing our thoughts and beliefs to be more positive can serve to change our lives for the better. One of the most important ways to do this is to learn to love and expect the very best for yourself—not in a selfish, narcissistic way, but in a very deep and loving way. I highly recommend exploring Louise Hay's books and trying out mirror work as well. Indeed, because of her recommendation of the New Thought movement, both Steve and I went on to participate in various Center for Spiritual Living (CSL) communities.[8]

Interestingly, the importance of developing self-love and self-compassion has recently become the foundation of a growing movement within modern psychology. If you are interested in learning more about it, go online and search for the term "self-compassion." You will find lots of books, workbooks, workshops, meditations, and other material.[9] There is also growing scientific evidence of the benefits of self-compassion practices. Happily, most of them can be done on your own at no cost.

The Sedona Method

Sometimes listening to your Astral Body and sending it all the loving words and compassion you can muster is still not enough. Although you may succeed in uncovering many of your subconscious patterns and beliefs, they may still haunt you. If so, you need to find a way to *release* (not suppress) them so that you can get beyond them.

One of the best ways I've found for doing so is called the *Sedona Method*.[10] Developed by Lester Levenson in the mid-1900s and now taught by his protégé Hale Dwoskin, the Sedona Method is comprised of a set of simple, yet surprisingly effective, techniques for releasing emotional patterns or beliefs. Like anything of this nature, however, you must earnestly engage with it in order for it to benefit you.

Unlike therapies with similar goals that involve the Physical Body (which I will discuss in the next section), the Sedona Method is purely a thought-based process. The most basic technique goes something like this. Suppose that you would like to release a specific emotional pattern—for instance, anger at your friend Sam. The first step is to welcome that emotion. Fully feel and welcome your feeling of anger at Sam. Next, ask yourself the question, "Can I release my anger at Sam?" Your answer may be yes or no. Often it's no, and that's fine. Next, ask yourself "*Would* I release my anger at Sam?" (Alternatively, you might use the phrase "Am I *willing* to release my anger at Sam?") Often the answer to this is yes, because a "no" answer would imply that you want to stay angry at Sam forever. But even if your answer is still no, move on to the last step. Ask yourself, "*When?*"

Somehow, saying this last word can bring a feeling of release, even if it's small. You might cry a bit, let out a sigh, or feel a subtle shift inside. Then repeat the process a few times. Often the emotional pattern will weaken as you do so.

Naturally, the Sedona Method involves a lot more than just these four steps. For instance, Hale Dwoskin's excellent book, *The Sedona Method*,[10] delves into the various layers that underlie stuck emotional patterns. Usually, they boil down to four basic desires: for approval, control, security, or separation (or its opposite, oneness). The process of uncovering the desires that underlie a stuck emotion often reveals subconscious feelings and beliefs that go way back to early childhood. Once revealed, you can then work on releasing these feelings and beliefs.

I have found the Sedona Method to be truly life-transforming. My first intense efforts at utilizing it were directed at solving my chronic insomnia. As I read Dwoskin's book, I journaled every step of the way and engaged in every exercise. The process took me an entire year! But I can honestly say that doing so uncovered and released many patterns, which ultimately *did* relieve my insomnia. Of course, I always have more inner work to do—as we all do. Luckily, I have continued to find the

Sedona Method to be one of my most effective tools. And much to my surprise, other members of my family are now engaging with the Sedona Method too.

Since writing his book, Hale Dwoskin has gone on to expand and modify many of the techniques that comprise the Sedona Method. For example, the basic formula for a release has changed over time, though the old formula described above is still a great place to start. He teaches many workshops and there is a lot of free material online.

Finally, another body of work that has similarities to the Sedona Method is Michael Singer's work on surrendering to what *is* and trusting in the flow of life. I highly recommend his books and meditations, and especially his fascinating book *The Surrender Experiment*.[11]

Core Transformation

Also similar to the Sedona Method is a technique called *Core Transformation*.[12] The key assumption underlying this method is that the unconscious mind (the Astral Body) is inherently benevolent; it is always trying to communicate with you and protect you.

The basic process of Core Transformation is simple. Start with any issue that has been troubling you, settle into a light meditative state, and ask your Astral Body, "What do you want? What are you trying to tell me?" After you receive an answer, ask, "If you had this (the desired thing), how would you feel? What would you then want?" Repeat this process until you reach some core state or need—usually something like peace, love, etc. Then feel that state deeply.

Interestingly and somewhat paradoxically, this process alone can bring a quick sense of relief. Moreover, if you can recall and bring up your final core state when you are feeling distressed, the result can be similar. I have only limited experience with Core Transformation and have experimented with it on some personal fears and physical aches and pains. I have found it to be quickly enlightening, and it allows me to better understand the root of an issue at hand. In essence, Core Transformation, like many of the methods in this section, helps to bring unconscious needs and wants into conscious awareness. As a result, the Astral Body feels heard and relief can follow. Those who are interested in learning more or would like to find a Core Transformation practitioner can visit coretransformation.org.

Family Constellation Therapy

Another fascinating and quite mysterious astral level therapy is *Family Constellation Therapy*.[13] I heard about this type of work many years ago at a homeopathy workshop, but I didn't experience it until I got a small, yet potent, dose of it at a retreat in 2023. Family Constellation Therapy directly utilizes the phenomenon of psychic connection and synchronicity to heal.

The person undergoing Constellation Therapy is usually assisted not only by a facilitator therapist, but also by helper volunteers who act as *surrogates*. Usually, each of the surrogates represents a family member (alive or dead), but sometimes they represent concepts like "yes" or "no." During a session, surrogates let themselves be "taken over" by their roles and move and act as directed by their intuition.

My own experience with this therapy lasted only fifteen minutes but left me so emotionally affected that I needed to change my clothes afterward; I was drenched in sweat! In my case, I was seeking healing so that I could finally fully accept my move from California to South Carolina. At the time of this experience, we had lived in our new home for about six months. Steve had fully embraced the move, but I still had feelings of sadness and anger. The two surrogates who volunteered to help me represented "yes" (embracing the move) and "no" (resistance to the move). During the session, each of us moved about in the room as our intuition directed us, with the facilitator asking us questions that we answered. By the end of the session, I was weeping on my hands and knees! But afterwards, I felt much more relaxed and at peace with what Steve and I had undergone over the preceding few years.

CONNECT WITH THE ASTRAL BODY VIA THE PHYSICAL BODY

So far, I have talked about connecting with your Astral Body primarily through your thoughts and emotions. But your Physical Body can also be an important conduit for reaching out to this part of you. After all, as I've already stressed, your Astral Body is highly impressed by input from your physical senses and actions. In this section, I'll discuss a variety of therapies that make use of this fact by co-mingling Astral Body work with strategies that stimulate the Physical Body in some way.

EFT (Emotional Freedom Technique) and TFT (Thought Field Therapy)

About twenty years ago, I heard about a new way of dealing with difficult emotions called Emotional Freedom Technique (EFT).[14] Popularized by Gary Craig, author of the highly popular book *The EFT Manual*, the basic technique involves tapping on a sequence of acupuncture points while repeating a phrase of the form, "Even though '*description of the problem*,' I deeply and completely accept myself." For example, "Even though I have this headache, I deeply and completely accept myself" or "Even though I'm having an anxiety attack, I deeply and completely accept myself." It is easy to see how these statements are related to the self-compassion techniques described earlier.

Intrigued by what I heard and read about EFT, I went to Craig's EFT website emofree.com (also check out eftinternational.org), and I tried to utilize the technique on my own, using the free online video instructions. I did meet with some success and added EFT to my self-help tool-kit. Then, in 2005, I began experiencing problems with dizziness (caused by menopause) that had become limiting for me. Without warning, a wave of dizziness would hit me, especially if I was stressed or tense. Sometimes it would even occur while I was driving, especially if it was in fast, dense traffic. Although I tried EFT on my own for this problem, I couldn't alleviate it. Eventually, I decided to find an EFT practitioner and made an appointment with Ellen Miller, who had an office nearby. Ultimately, this fortuitous step led to many significant changes in my life.

During my sessions with Ellen, I began by briefly describing problems I was experiencing. Then we began tapping. Sometimes Ellen tapped on me, and sometimes I tapped on myself. Although she used a somewhat different sequence of tapping points and movements than the ones described in Craig's book, I quickly found that one session of EFT was as effective as weeks or even months of psychotherapy. I also learned that an important aspect of EFT is discovering what arises as a *result* of the tapping procedure.

For example, suppose that you begin by tapping on the fact that you have a headache. After doing so, you may experience an emotion, thought, or a new physical sensation—say, a clenched jaw. After you tap on the experience of jaw tension, you might suddenly remember an interaction with your boss and how angry you felt. Then, after you tap on "angry at my boss," things will likely go even deeper—for instance, recalling a difficult experience in childhood. You keep going deeper and deeper with the tapping process until you can't find anything else.

In essence, EFT is a way to uncover the underlying root of a problem, buried deep within the subconscious Astral Body. The process can be amazingly quick compared to, say, conventional talk psychotherapy. And like the Sedona Method, it can be extremely effective at releasing feelings if used repeatedly. Indeed, after only a few appointments with Ellen, my dizziness was greatly alleviated. I also found that if I did start to feel dizzy, tapping could stop the sensation pretty quickly.

Given the knowledge I gained from working with Ellen, I became more adept at applying EFT on my own. I even began to teach it to my immediate family. But one of the best things that happened was that I began to take a series of meditation and self-awareness classes with Ellen and her husband Gary Sherman. In fact, I would probably never have written this book or my preceding book, *Active Consciousness*, if I had not contacted Ellen so many years ago for help with EFT.

Since that time, I have become aware of a set of techniques that are similar to EFT called TFT—Thought Field Therapy. It turns out that the development of TFT preceded that of EFT, and that Gary Craig's formulation of EFT was essentially a simplified version of TFT that could be learned more easily. TFT does not use a single tapping procedure for all problems like EFT does. Instead, different tapping methods are utilized for different kinds of problems. There are many books available that teach TFT and some online reviewers claim that they find it to be more effective than EFT. One useful and insightful book that I have read is *Your Power to Heal* by Henry Grayson, Ph.D.,[15] which discusses TFT, EFT, and other similar techniques that clear energy blockages. If you are interested in exploring a tapping therapy, buy a book about EFT or TFT, perhaps find a certified practitioner, and try it out for yourself.

EMDR (Eye Movement Desensitization and Reprocessing)

Another method in this category is EMDR or Eye Movement Desensitization and Reprocessing.[16] Developed in the late 1980s and 1990s as a way of dealing with trauma, EMDR is typically utilized by psychotherapists as part of their work with clients. In fact, I went to a therapist in the late 1980s who used this procedure during some of my appointments. At the time, I didn't know why or what she was doing, but I now realize that she was utilizing EMDR. First, she asked me to think about a traumatic event I had been describing. While I did so, she asked me to follow her finger with my eyes. Then she quickly and repeatedly moved it back and forth in front of my eyes, from right to left and back again.

The idea behind EMDR is that the physical brain stimulation triggered by back-and-forth eye movements creates a phenomenon akin to what occurs during rapid eye movement (REM) sleep. EMDR therapists believe that this brain stimulation helps a client to process and gain insight into their difficult memories and feelings, thereby allowing them to heal. EMDR therapists also find that the procedure can accelerate insight and self-awareness more quickly and effectively than pure talk therapy. Interestingly, both EFT and TFT often incorporate various eye movements too. Similar eye movements are also utilized during the induction phase of hypnotherapy.

TRE (Trauma Release Exercises)

Another movement therapy that has become an important part of my life is TRE, sometimes called "shaking."[17] This therapy is the brainchild of Dr. Peter Levine. He noticed that after wild zebras in Africa survived the trauma of a lion attack, they would go into the bush and engage in intense body shaking. Afterwards, they seemed relaxed and rejoined the herd.

The underlying idea of TRE is that trauma is literally stored in the body and that induced body shaking helps to dislodge and release it. It can be used to relieve trauma that is acknowledged consciously as well as buried subconscious trauma. As I described in the introduction, when the COVID vaccination campaign began, my husband Steve and I slowly became more and more ostracized by friends and family because we chose not to be vaccinated. That alone was traumatic, but as it became clear that our status as pariahs necessitated our leaving California entirely, the trauma ran even deeper. I was angry, anxious, sad, and confused. At about the same time, I learned about TRE and decided to find a practitioner. Luckily, I found someone who worked online and did not judge my vaccination status.

My experience with TRE was intense and deeply therapeutic. Each session began with a discussion of what was going on for me and my feelings about it. Then I engaged in several rounds of shaking, each lasting a minute or two. I laid on a mat on the floor and after some preparatory movements, my legs started to shake. As time went on, it became easier to let it all go and shake my arms and head too and even scream and cry. I knew that the process was complete when a calm inner knowing came over me; the sensation felt like I had become more connected to my wise Causal Body. Although I felt somewhat agitated for about a half-hour after each session, it definitely resulted in healing for me.

When Steve and I hit the road in search of our new home, I started using TRE every night to release the stress of our voyage and to fall asleep in yet another hotel room. I still perform it each night after I get into bed, even if I feel fine consciously, because the shaking process can uncover and release little tensions of the day that have become unconscious. I highly recommend learning TRE and incorporating it into your daily health regimen. Why let issues build up? Release them as they occur. To find out more and find a practitioner, visit traumaprevention.com.

Breathwork, Sweat Lodges, Ecstatic Dance, Sound, and Plant Medicine

In order to contact your Astral Body, sometimes you simply need to get out of your everyday monkey mind and enter a completely different state of consciousness. Of course, meditation has the same goal. So does hypnotherapy. Another way to enter an altered state is to exert an unusual force upon the Physical Body. That is why people engage in various breathwork therapies, undergo extreme heat in a sweat lodge ceremony, tax their bodies during ecstatic dancing, put on earphones and listen to vibrations specifically designed to shift their brain waves, or take a plant medicine that carries them into a new state of perception. I'll review some of these methods in this section, though there are hundreds of techniques out there. Indeed, every culture on Earth has its own.

Among the many types of breathwork therapy are Holotropic breathwork, Rebirthing breathwork, Clarity breathwork, Biodynamic breathwork, and Integrative breathwork.[18] The idea is that by consciously altering your breathing pattern, you also alter your state of mind and emotions. Many of these therapies are rooted in Eastern wisdom practices like Yoga and Tai Chi. Some also integrate the use of music and art to aid in the awareness-shifting process. A sweat lodge, in contrast, is usually associated with Native American traditions. Unlike a simple sauna (which can also be healing), a sweat lodge is an extended ceremonial experience, usually accompanied by drumming, chanting, and meditation.

Another way to dramatically shift your state is through movement. The whirling dervishes of the Sufi tradition in Turkey, for example, engage in a specific and prolonged twirling dance that puts them into a trance-like state. Spiritual teacher G.I. Gurdieff,[1] also from the Middle East, developed a variety of transformative movement exercises in the early 1900s with the same goal. In addition, he emphasized that our everyday postures—the way we hold our bodies—can not only tell others something about us, but can affect our state of awareness.

Today's practitioners of Ecstatic Dance[19] also use movement to change their state of consciousness. You may be able to join such events if you live in an urban area. The basic idea behind them is to simply let it all hang out and permit your instincts and feelings to guide you as you move, dance, and interact with others for several hours, all while listening to powerful, rhythmic music. Of course, people all over the world experience a version of this at rock concerts and raves.

And then there is the use of music and sound itself. Just as eye movements can pop your brain into an altered state of consciousness, so can some sounds. I already mentioned this in Chapter 15 when I discussed the work of the Monroe Institute; the institute even claims to have discovered sound protocols that trigger the states induced by plant medicines.

While I'm on the subject, it is quite likely that you are already aware of the mind-altering effects of smokable and ingestible plants, ranging from cannabis to the more potent ayahuasca, peyote, and others. There are also modern chemical equivalents like Ecstasy (MDMA) and LSD. All of these substances directly affect the brain so that perceptions are altered in a variety of ways. Whether the effects are beneficial, however, can vary. Personally, I would exercise caution, because many plant medicines have been known to trigger psychoses, especially if used repeatedly or by susceptible individuals. Certainly, one could argue that the social revolutions of the 1960s could be partially attributed to the widespread use of cannabis and LSD. Indeed, writers like Graham Hancock[20] suggest that shamanic practitioners of prehistoric times were also utilizing plant medicines, and as a result, shifted the consciousness of all of humanity, ultimately leading to quantum leaps in human evolution.

Shamanism

Some people derisively call them "witch doctors." But the truth is, *true* shamans are perhaps the most powerful healers we have among us. They are men and women trained to heal on every level, from the physical to the causal. Most shamans use many of the techniques already described—sweat lodges, dance, drumming, rattles, and plant medicines—to shift their own and their patients' awareness. But perhaps their greatest area of expertise is on the astral level. A true shaman, like a medium, has the ability to perceive and operate within the astral realm.

Interestingly, shamans aren't like Western practitioners who go to a school and learn a set of healing skills. Instead, they are called to it and are recognized by others as individuals with inherent abilities. Usually, shamans undergo a severe initiation process that includes a near-death experience. And because of their abilities and self-imposed trials, shamans are usually revered and sometimes feared.

A shaman knows all about the Astral Body and the fact that verbal suggestions and rituals powerfully affect it. When a "witch doctor" puts on a frightening mask and does a healing dance, they know that this can heal a patient because the Astral Body ultimately controls the Physical Body. And when they put a "hex" on someone, they understand that this *can* have a negative effect—just like a nocebo message from an unwitting doctor. Too bad doctors don't know what shamans know!

But a truly powerful shaman can do a lot more than make suggestions and perform rituals. They can figure out what's really going on within a patient's Astral Body. For instance, they might be able to see harmful astral spirits and release their influence. Sadly, evil shamans might use their power to *create* such attachments in order to kill or injure someone. Some shamans utilize their psychic powers to witness past lives that may be causing undue influence, or to predict possible futures to be wary of. They might also be able to read the collective astral energies of a group of people and conduct ceremonies that achieve the healing of a family or tribe.

While many shamans operating in the Western world are hucksters, some really do have abilities. I once had a reading from a Siberian shaman who told me about one of my incarnations—from the past or the future, I do not know. She told me that I had been a scientist trying to develop an unusual energy device with a group of colleagues. One day, while I was away from my laboratory, my collaborators were brutally murdered by people trying to undermine our work. As the shaman told me this rather far-fetched tale, I began sobbing uncontrollably. I had never imagined or dreamed of such a scenario, but I instinctively knew it was true. It could also explain the pervasive sense of guilt I've carried around since I was a little girl. In fact, my mother told me that I used to go around the house saying "It's all my fault" when I was three-years old.

Another healer who could read past lives told me about a similar past-life scenario. In this one, I was an orthodox priest in Eastern Europe in the 1600s or 1700s. Maybe this past life explains why I've always been drawn to monastic music, like Gregorian chants or the music of Hildegard von Bingen. The healer told me that as an important clergy leader in my town, I was close to members of the Jewish community living there. Unfortunately, the Jews in the town were massacred when I was away travelling. When I (the priest) returned, I felt terribly guilty that I had not been there to stop the carnage. Once again, I sobbed uncontrollably when I was told this story. But the healer reassured me that the massacre victims did not blame me and were grateful for everything I had done for them. Once again, something about this story rang true for me. And both of these incarnational memories, retrieved from the astral realm, had a powerful healing effect upon me.

There is so much more about the practice of shamanism that is beyond the scope of this book. If you are interested, I encourage you to learn more through reading or perhaps seek out a recommended shaman for yourself. As I will discuss in the next two chapters, such practitioners can be also skilled at working at the mental and causal levels. Don't forget—the higher up you go within the energetic realms, the more encompassing and powerful the potential healing effects can be.

CHAPTER 17

ン

WE ARE WILLFUL, THINKING, MEANING-FULL BEINGS

When it comes to the Mental Body and the mental realm in general, it's all about thought and meaning. Our Mental Body is what enables us to think, calculate, plan, and be rational. It is also the seat of the power of will.

Lest you still have confusion about it, know that your Mental Body is *not* your brain. Yes, our brains are very important tools that our Mental Bodies utilize while we are in physical form. If a brain is atrophied due to neurological disease, it isn't able to do much calculating, just as nothing will appear on your TV if it is broken. Even so, the Mental Body will still be there and will continue to be present until death. Also remember that the Mental Body is not where your emotions originate, nor does it store your memories. That is the job of the Astral Body.

You might think of the Mental Body as a computer without much memory storage but lots of abilities. Think about the stereotype of the absent-minded math professor. They may be a wiz at abstract thought but cannot remember appointments or where their car keys are. Such a person may also tend to be disconnected from their bodily functions, not like to exercise, and can't relate emotionally to other people. In other words, they have a highly developed Mental Body, but don't have much going on in the physical and astral realms.

UNTANGLE YOUR PERCEPTION OF YOUR HIGHER BODIES

It is actually quite enlightening to learn how to disentangle the distinct perceptions you are picking up from your Physical, Etheric, Astral, Mental, and Causal Bodies. Your Physical Body picks up information by utilizing the senses we are all familiar with: taste, touch, hearing, vision, and smell. Your Etheric Body senses subtle vibrations and energies at a deeper level. Your Astral Body feels your emotions, picks up psychic perceptions, and stores and retrieves past memories and beliefs. It is then your Mental Body that does your thinking, sends its dictums to the Astral Body, and receives inspiration and insight from the greater mental and causal realms.

Unfortunately, most of the time, we tend to confuse our feelings, thoughts, and sensations and can suffer as a result. Learning to distinguish between these things and skillfully integrate them together is what my teacher Gary Sherman focuses on in his workshops. It's a skill he calls *perceptual integration.*[1] For example, if you can separate a feeling from a thought, you can more easily detach your emotions about a difficult subject if you are trying to reason about it. Similarly, if you can detach your emotional feelings from bodily sensations, you can become more adept at realizing that, for instance, your stomachache is actually arising from anger rather than from a bad meal. This could then enable you to cure your stomach pain by releasing that anger. Interestingly, it can go the other way too. That is, by simply relaxing your stomach, you may find that you also release your anger. Try it! It can be quite surprising.

Happily, once you've learned to distinguish between these inputs from different parts of your complete Self, your life will become much easier to navigate. Instead of finding yourself lost in a jumble of confusing information, everything is put into its proper place and a greater sense of calm can be achieved. You can also more easily hone your ability to perceive with each of your bodies.

So let's get back to the Mental Body. What exactly is it all about?

Yes, it thinks and is conscious. It forms conclusions from memories of the past that it retrieves from the Astral Body, and it instructs the Astral Body to store its conclusions as new beliefs. It helps you to plan your day and to navigate your way home from work. It strategizes your various efforts, based on past and present information available to it and the possible futures it projects. The Mental Body may also utilize psychic perceptions received from the Astral Body and wisdom gleaned from the Causal Body.

The Mental Body can receive information from the larger mental realm too. In fact, that's how many inspirations occur. When a scientist, musician, or artist has an "Aha!" moment that seems to come out of nowhere (that is, it does not arise from logical reasoning or past experience), it might very well be a message sent to their Mental Body from the larger mental realm. Maybe that's why scientific breakthroughs are often discovered independently at the same time. These new inspirations may literally be bubbles of information within the mental realm that finally penetrate and become perceived by the people who are ready for them or ask for them. Of course, inspirational thoughts may be arising from the causal realm too.

MEANING

This brings me to the next and perhaps most important quality of the mental realm: the primacy of meaning. Remember our previous discussions about synchronicity? Synchronicities are *meaningful* coincidences. For example, suppose you are thinking about something or feeling a certain emotion, and suddenly, something with a similar or connected meaning appears in your physical world. That's a synchronicity.

I like to think of a specific "meaning" as a vibrational form or pattern that can appear in all of the realms—from physical to causal. Moreover, I believe that things with similar "meaning vibrations" tend to appear simultaneously in time and space. If I'm right, then synchronicity may be a phenomenon caused by a fundamental vibrational law of nature.

As an example, suppose your Mental Body receives a new insight from the mental realm. Some representation of this insight may then synchronistically appear in your outer life. It might be an image you see, a sound you hear, a person you run into, or a series of events. Or it might be received as a dream. Often, these synchronistic events appear as *symbols*—shapes or occurrences that are culturally associated with particular meanings. That's why dreams are often permeated with symbolic content whose meaning conveys the dream's message. And once you notice a synchronicity, your conscious Mental Body can use its rational thinking ability to decipher and understand it.

Finally, I also believe that the co-occurrence of similar vibrations in time and space are not strictly a passive aspect of nature. *Synchronicity can also be intentionally and actively utilized as a tool.* That's what the process of manifestation and creation is all about, abilities that I will discuss at length in the next chapter. It is also a key subject of my second book *Active Consciousness.* These powers are the domain of the Causal Body.

THE POWER OF WILL

Meaning may actually be the secret sauce that underlies a key feature of humanity: *the power of will* or *will power*. In fact, will power may be the greatest power we possess. It is the force that enables our determination, intention, and the creative power of the Causal Body. In particular, the Mental Body thinks and decides what it wishes to achieve in terms of meaning, and then uses its will power to deliver that wish to the Causal Body for creation.

Perhaps you are familiar with Victor Frankl's renowned and life-transforming book, *Man's Search for Meaning*.[2] Frankl was a promising young psychiatrist in Austria when he was rounded up by the Nazis and sent to a series of concentration camps during World War II. At the time, he had just completed a manuscript for a book that emphasized the primacy of meaning in human life. His ideas were in direct opposition to those of his mentor Sigmund Freud, who emphasized pleasure as the prime human motivator. Little did Frankl know that the next phase of his life would serve as a proving ground for his new theory.

After he was captured, Frankl tried to hide his manuscript within the lining of his coat. But soon he found himself, like all of the other Jewish inmates around him, stripped of every physical vestige of his former self and subjugated to unspeakable horror. The first half of *Man's Search for Meaning* recounts Frankl's experiences in the camps. It especially focuses on what he learned, filtered through his perspective as a psychiatrist, and is truly a fascinating read. As one might expect, the dire circumstances within the concentration camps led to all kinds of human behaviors—from the most base and cruel (with the Nazis choosing the most violent and amoral inmates to police and brutalize the others), to lofty acts of self-sacrifice, nobility, and integrity.

Frankl managed to survive his internments at four different camps, including the infamous Auschwitz, through a mixture of luck, ingenuity, and the fact that being a medical doctor had its uses to the Nazis. One of the primary things he took away from his experiences was the realization that the people who tended to survive were those who found something to live for. Usually, these survivors found some form of meaning, purpose, or vision for *after* the war, despite the hopeless circumstances and horrors that were going on all around them each day. Indeed, Frankl credits his own survival to his determination to someday rewrite and publish his book. Even during a nearly fatal case of typhus, he kept trying to write snippets on any shred of paper he could find.

Frankl also noticed a common pattern among those who died. If an inmate suddenly refused to get up out of bed in the morning and started smoking a prized cigarette they had hidden, they would most likely die within a couple of days. These people had simply given up and had decided that they no longer had any reason to live. In fact, they *wanted* to die. Because of this phenomenon, Frankl tried to provide psychotherapy to his fellow inmates, encouraging them to find some kind of meaning that could sustain them. After the war, the various strategies he developed blossomed into a new branch of psychotherapy called *logotherapy*, which I will discuss in greater detail later on in this chapter.

Of course, you don't need to be confined to a concentration camp in order to witness the truth of Frankl's ideas. It's quite common to see someone unexpectedly die when they can no longer find meaning in their life—for example, after a spouse dies. On the flip side, finding meaning and purpose can enable someone to survive even the most difficult circumstances. The life story of Supreme Court Justice Ruth Bader Ginsburg provides an excellent illustration. This tiny woman was a veritable powerhouse of determination. Despite her age and multiple bouts with cancer, she continued to inspire everyone with her rigorous workout regimens and long work hours. She was absolutely driven by the meaning she derived from her work.

DISEASE WITHIN THE MENTAL BODY

So what does disease within the Mental Body look like? How do we get out of sync with this quintessentially human part of ourselves? What causes our rational thought processes to be undermined? What can we do when we can no longer find meaning in our lives or muster the will to achieve something? How can we heal our Mental Body and even increase its power to become more aware of synchronicities and insights?

To be certain, disease within the physical brain can wreak havoc upon our basic reasoning and planning abilities. We are all too familiar these days with diseases like Alzheimer's, which assault the brain and other parts of the Physical Body. When we are incarnated into physical form, our Mental Body needs our Physical Body to operate effectively in the physical world. In my opinion, most of the increasingly common neurological diseases today are being driven by environmental causes like poor food and diet, toxic chemicals and pesticides, electromagnetic pollution, and the ill-advised overuse of modern drugs, including vaccines.

Of course, the Astral Body can also play a part in undermining Mental Body functioning. Even conventional scientists agree that chronic fear, depression, and other forms of emotional stress can literally rob the brain of its ability to perform rational thought processes. Panic, anger, and fear all cloud our judgment. With a never-ending stream of media that amplify such emotions and deluge our impressionable Astral Bodies with images, sounds, and words, it's easy to see why so many people are having a hard time getting their rational minds in gear and focusing on finding meaning.

So what can we do? The first step, as always, is to start by cleaning things up—from the physical level upward. That means finding ways to eat and sleep better, eliminate EMFs as much as possible, and minimize the influence of environmental toxins and drugs. We also need to become aware of and avoid the fear-mongering within our culture and admit that what we now accept as "normal" is actually creating ill health. Next, we can employ etheric therapies like homeopathy and acupuncture to bolster our resistance to these assaults. We also need to work hard on uncovering and releasing our emotional obstacles and turning down the volume of the media that trigger unhelpful emotions.

Finally, there is work we can do directly within the mental realm. The rest of this chapter will focus on a variety of tools and therapies of this kind that can help us to find meaning, increase our will power, and invigorate our ability to be inspired.

SIGNS AND CAUTIONS FOR THE MENTAL REALM

Let's begin by considering various signs and symptoms that may indicate you have a problem within your Mental Body:

- Lack of will and will power.

- A decreased ability to use the imagination or to be inspired by anything.

- Creative blocks.

- Difficulty with reasoning.

- Mental fog.

- Lack of dreams.

- An inability to find meaning in life. Existential angst.

- Ennui.

- Addictions that are used as an avoidance or coping mechanism.

Of course, many of these symptoms can also be signs of trouble in the Physical, Etheric, and Astral Bodies. My advice is to address those areas first, in order to determine if the problem really *does* lie in your Mental Body. For example, poor sleep can lead to difficulties with reasoning. Lack of exercise and movement, which can result in poor blood circulation, can then lead to mental fog. Havoc in the gut or heart can affect the brain and the rest of the body. Emotional depression can lead to a loss of will power and ennui. Addiction can be a coping mechanism of the Astral Body, especially if your parents had similar problems.

But if you have already addressed these things, and in particular, if you still feel like life no longer has any meaning for you, it's time to address your problems directly at the mental level. Most tools and therapies within this realm are based on using your powerful mind and its thoughts—that is, your Mental Body itself. But, you may ask, how can mere thoughts heal you? Because your Mental Body is the boss of your Astral Body and therefore can have a tremendous effect on your Etheric and Physical Bodies too. That's why therapies that focus on the mind alone can create cures of all kinds—even physical ones.

But be forewarned: your powerful mind *can* be a clever adversary. It may try to avoid and elude your efforts, especially if it has already convinced itself that it's a good idea to have a particular problem. For this reason, it can be helpful to enlist the help of a therapist. As always, try to find a reputable one—someone you can trust and feel comfortable with.

MENTALLY-BASED THERAPIES

I've grouped the approaches and strategies below into three categories based on their primary focus—the past, the present, or the future.

1. *Look back: Apply your mind to gain a deeper understanding of your past.*
   Therapies in this category include traditional psychotherapy and newer psychological clarification methods like Byron Katie's "The Work." I'll also discuss techniques for becoming more aware of habitual thought processes and behaviors.

2. *In the present moment, look more deeply within and without: Apply your mind in order to notice, decode, and gain greater access to information arriving from the mental realm.*

 Techniques include meditation, noticing and decoding synchronicities or other signs that may be providing information to you, dream interpretation, and working with a shaman. Another method called *Logosynthesis* (not related to Logotherapy) is a word-based process that literally instructs the Mental Body (and other energy bodies) to release stored packets of harmful meaning that are harbored within it.

3. *Look forward: Apply your mind to find new meaning in your life and visualize what you want to create in the future.*

 As mentioned earlier, after World War II, psychiatrist Victor Frankl created a new meaning-focused branch of psychotherapy called *Logotherapy* that fits into this category.

Look Back

I have already discussed psychotherapy in Chapter 16. Although one goal of this form of treatment is to contact the (subconscious) Astral Body, by and large it tends to be focused on cultivating greater self-understanding within the Mental Body. That's why psychotherapy typically involves a lot of discussion about how experiences in the past shape who we are today. The idea is that if we can understand family issues, childhood traumas, work and relationship conflicts, and other patterns that affect us, we can learn to navigate our current and future lives more gracefully. In other words, by taking a rational and objective look at ourselves, we can not only find clarity, but also provide better direction and consolation to our Astral Body, and by extension, to our Etheric and Physical Bodies too.

For instance, suppose that you have developed an addiction to alcohol as a way of avoiding confrontation with others. By working with a therapist or through introspection, you might be able to admit to yourself that you *are* addicted and are using it as an avoidance strategy. You may also remember that a parent did the same thing, or that you've used other forms of addiction in the past for the same purpose—say, compulsive shopping or overeating. By gaining mental awareness and clarity around the issue, you are then enabled to form the intent and will to notice yourself engaging in this behavior and change it.

Psychotherapy can also help patients to look back on past trauma and reframe it so that it holds a less negative or even a positive charge. For example, when I was a child, I witnessed a few incidents of family violence that haunted me for years. As many children in such situations do, I found a way to blame myself for these events. The result was a lifelong emotional habit of guilt and anxiety. However, by looking back on these events from a more rational, adult perspective, I have come to realize and to gradually *believe* that these events were not my fault. Achieving this was harder than you might think because my guilt habit was so deeply ingrained. Luckily, after a lot of internal work, I was able to reframe my traumatic memories by focusing on the fact that, even as a little girl, I tried to stop the violence and even physically attempted to defend the person being attacked. In other words, I now choose to remember that I was *courageous* and even did some good. This has served to defuse the trauma considerably for me.

All of this underscores an important point: the Mental Body is a powerful, objective, and rational vehicle for noticing patterns. Many of the problems embedded within our Astral Bodies—especially worrying, anxiety, sadness, anger, guilt, and complaining—are simply habits we've stopped noticing. These emotional habits may also be ingrained as brain patterns. That's why breaking free from a habit—from a physical one like smoking to an emotional habit like anxiety—can not only be difficult, but somehow feel weird or wrong. To overcome this, we need our rational Mental Body to help us realize that these feelings are simply habits that *can* be changed. It can also help us to notice them when they arise and prompt us to choose, with intent and will, not to engage in them anymore.

The process of first *noticing* and then *changing* is also a strategy used by many behavioral therapies. Studies have shown that by catching a habit and engaging in a new replacement behavior for a period of three weeks, each of us can effectively break an unconscious habitual cycle. However, engaging in this kind of therapy requires your Mental Body to first realize that something is wrong and to adopt the goal of noticing and breaking the habit.

Another powerful Mental Body therapy is "The Work" made popular by author Byron Katie. Katie was a depressed addict wallowing in personal dysfunction and living in a half-way house when she had a breakthrough. Suddenly she realized that many of the beliefs that were driving her behavior simply weren't true or weren't true anymore. In other words, her Mental Body got in sync with what *is*. Indeed, perhaps these insights were delivered to her from the greater mental realm. Now, Katie understood that engaging with her erroneous beliefs was completely self-defeating, and that other beliefs she held were projections or other kinds of reversals of thought. Her rational Mental Body had suddenly gained insight into the situation, which enabled her to break free from her self-imposed prison of astral beliefs and emotions. Eventually, she went on to write about her experience and insights, helping countless others.

I highly recommend reading one of Byron Katie's books and engaging with her method. You might begin with her first book, *Loving What Is*.[3] This book has had a profound influence on everyone in my family. In it, Katie outlines the four simple questions that comprise her method. Why not try it out now? If a belief is causing you anguish, ask yourself:

1. Is it true?

2. Can you absolutely know that it is true?

3. How does it make you feel when you believe that thought?

4. What would you be like without that thought or belief?

The final fifth step is to perform what Katie calls a "turn around"—essentially, one of many possible reversals of the belief. For example, if you believe "Joe hates me," then one reversal might be "Joe doesn't hate me." Another is "I hate Joe." The trick is to find a thought reversal that resonates with you. When you do, it can lead to profound insight and relief.

Loving What Is also includes many real-life examples of people doing "The Work" at Katie's workshops. A few years ago, I attended a short workshop at which Katie led us through a series of exercises. One was particularly profound for me as well as for my husband Steve when I told him about it later that evening. The exercise involved recalling your earliest memory from childhood. Then a variety of questions were posed to tease out what that particular memory means in a larger sense. Both Steve and I found that our first childhood memory did indeed echo some core elements of who we became later in life.

In my case, I remembered that when I was about two years old, I got out of my crib, opened a closed cupboard door, and climbed up the drawers to reach the top shelf. My mother then entered the room, panicked, and scolded me—understandable from an adult perspective. However, I felt crestfallen and disappointed that she did not recognize and praise me for my amazing and ingenious accomplishment. The insight I gained from this memory? That it reflected a lifelong theme in my relationship with my mother—of feeling she did not recognize me for who I am, or acknowledge my accomplishments. This led to deep feelings of disappointment and hurt. But what was *really* true? Today, I understand that she suffered from mild depression, that she often didn't know how to relate to me, and that she was possibly intimidated by me. Happily, when she was in her late 80's and 90's, we finally discussed these issues and resolved them before her death.

In the Present Moment, Look More Deeply Within and Without

As I've discussed throughout this book, the mental realm can be a magical place that holds information for us—if we choose to access it. One of the ways this information can appear is in the form of synchronistic co-occurrences of meaningfully related events. By using our skillful Mental Body, we can hone our ability to *notice* and *decode* these events when they appear in our inner and outer worlds.

A key method for accessing and enhancing this skill is meditation. When we meditate, we clear away our emotional reactions as well as busy and distracting thoughts. With a quieter mind, we can then open ourselves up to receive new and meaningful information. This was the message of Chapter 4, "The Box."

For example, try this out the next time you meditate. After your mind is quiet, pose a specific question to your Mental Body. You might ask for guidance in solving a technical problem, for creative inspiration, or for deeper understanding about a perplexing issue. The answer might arrive as words, images, or even as a sound within. It could also appear later as an event, dream, or physical sign. If you need to, ask your Mental Body for help in decoding these answers.

Another way to work with your Mental Body is to ask it to notice important insights and synchronicities more often. The fact is, they happen every day! We tend to gloss over them and ignore them, but the more you make an effort to notice these missives from the mental realm, the more often they will occur. In other words, just by *asking* and *noticing*, you create a foundation for better communication with this part of yourself.

But how do you know if something is a genuine communication from the mental realm and not just the result of wishful thinking or a conventional thought process? The answer is that this information doesn't *feel* like it was reasoned out. Instead, it just popped into awareness. It is also usually accompanied by feelings like joy, elation, energy, and a sense that something significant has happened.

Some psychotherapists can help you with this process. Or you can try to find a genuine shaman who is skilled at communicating with the mental realm and is able to ask for information and interpret it. They can also help you to enter into a trance state, in which this kind of information can more easily be accessed. Just be certain that the shaman you are working with is legitimate and has integrity.

Another present-moment meaning-based technique is *Logosynthesis*. (The term "logos" means "logic," "message," or "reason"—all aspects of the Mental Body.) Developed by Dutch/Swiss psychotherapist Dr. Willem Lammers, Logosynthesis is based on the idea that packets of meaning or "thought forms"—which you might think of as vibrational patterns—can literally be stored in your body. Unfortunately, counterproductive thought forms—negative energy packets—can create blockages. The method then uses word phrases to instruct the Mental Body to dislodge these thought forms, thereby freeing up energy and enabling a reconnection to life essence and purpose. You can learn more about Logosynthesis by going to logosynthesis.net or by reading Lammers' recent book, *Discover Logosynthesis: The Power of Words in Healing and Development.*[4]

Although the Logosynthesis method is very simple in concept, like all such therapies, there is a lot behind it. I first learned the basic technique during COVID and used it to release my anxiety about the disease. No doubt, harmful thought forms about COVID invaded the bodies of almost everyone on Earth, propagated by the ever-present media.

Since that time, I often use Logosynthesis to release negative thought forms in my body in order to prepare for sleep. First, I try to figure out which thought form I'd like to dislodge (it is often forgotten). Engaging in TRE shaking first (which I described in the last chapter) can be helpful in doing so. I then choose a simple phrase to denote the target thought form. Finally, I utilize the basic Logosynthesis formula provided below to release it. For example, during COVID, I used the phrase "COVID" to denote the thought form. Today, it might be something like "What '*so-and-so*' said to me" or about a disturbing video I had watched.

The basic Logosynthesis formula is comprised of three statements. (Note: '*target phrase*' denotes your targeted thought form.) Each statement should be said *out loud* (remember that doing so affects the Astral Body more powerfully), and after each one, take a few minutes to rest and reflect. During this period, various thoughts and sensations may come up. Once these dissipate, move on to the next statement. In my experience, at least one of these statements usually causes some kind of release within me—often accompanied by a sigh of relief.

1. "I retrieve all of my energy bound up in the energy field of '*target phrase*' in my physical, mental, and social system, in all representations of '*target phrase*' in my system, and in everything '*target phrase*' represents, and take it to the right place in my Self."

2. "I cancel the energy of '*target phrase*' on all frequencies, the frequencies of all its representations and of everything it represents, in all of my body and in all of my systems, dissolving it in pure white light."

3. "I retrieve all of my energy bound up in all my reactions to the energy field of '*target phrase*' in the field I'm living in, to all its representations and to everything it represents, and take it to the right place in my Self."

234 LIVING IN SYNCHRONY

Look Forward

As Victor Frankl so eloquently conveyed in his book *Man's Search for Meaning*,[1] when it comes to propelling humans forward, there is nothing as powerful as finding meaning and purpose. Unfortunately, as he also pointed out, more and more people in the modern world are plagued by the inability to do so. Feelings of meaninglessness and ennui have reached epidemic proportions today, even though so many people are doing quite well from a materialistic point of view.

Perhaps it is materialism itself, with its underlying assumption that humans are nothing more than biological robots, living in a random and fundamentally meaningless world, that is fueling this collective existential angst and despair. The symptoms are increasing every year: depression, anxiety, and a growing incidence of addictions of every kind—to alcohol, opioids and other drugs, shopping and the accumulation of material wealth, overeating, sex, and other distractions like texting, video, and social media. As Mattias Desmet so eloquently points out in his landmark book, *The Psychology of Totalitarianism*,[5] materialism and feelings of meaninglessness are the breeding ground for the emergence and embrace of totalitarianism, which we also see on the rise today, especially since COVID.

So how *can* we find meaning? Frankl claimed that there are three basic ways:

1. By accomplishing or doing something in the outer world;

2. By experiencing things like beauty, travel, learning, art, music, nature, and especially love;

3. Through *unavoidable* suffering, which can ennoble and teach the sufferer, test their courage, and challenge them to find meaning despite their suffering.

Certainly, the first method of finding meaning is the one recognized by most people. We all know that we can be driven forward in life by goals like striving to receive an education, building a home, succeeding in work, taking care of our families, and giving back to others through service. Unfortunately, modern society tends to devalue people who are no longer actively working or raising a family—especially the elderly. Instead, we should encourage older people to use the second method— that is, deriving meaning through experiences—for example, through travel, enjoying the arts, or engaging with the natural world. This will help them to become the wise elders that we can call upon in difficult times.

Of course, one thing that modern society certainly does *not* value is unavoidable suffering. In fact, we often shame and isolate sufferers, which only adds to their plight. Note, however, that suffering has to be *unavoidable* in order to provide meaning. If a person's suffering can be alleviated, not doing so is simply a symptom of masochism—an Astral Body affliction. And it is certainly not ennobling or meaningful for someone to wallow and indulge in their suffering or to use it to manipulate others.

So how can the meaning of *unavoidable* suffering be harnessed? The first step is to recognize that no matter what the circumstances, finding meaning is possible for every person. After all, as Frankl showed, if this can be done in the bowels of the Nazi concentration camps, it can be achieved by anyone. Rather than insulating ourselves from unavoidable sufferers so that we no longer have to be reminded that they exist, we should acknowledge and learn from their struggle, courage, triumphs, and emotional growth. By doing so, we can help them to cope better and to find meaning too.

Finding meaning is the purpose of Frankl's *Logotherapy*. He developed this form of treatment after his experiences during World War II. In essence, it is a type of psychotherapy based on the assumption that life *is* inherently meaningful (instead of inherently meaningless). Logotherapists believe that all people have a will and a need for meaning, and that finding meaning is always possible. Moreover, because what is meaningful is unique for each individual, logotherapists do not impose or suggest meaning to a client, but rather, try to help them discover it for themselves.

In addition to the basic Socratic method (asking and answering questions), logotherapists utilize two interesting techniques: *dereflection* and *paradoxical intention*. In dereflection, someone who is embroiled and fixated upon themself is encouraged to divert their attention outward onto something that is important to them. For example, if a person is obsessing about an emotional hurt, a logotherapist might encourage them to focus on education, exercise, or service.

The technique of *paradoxical intention* is fascinating to me because it parallels the homeopathic principle. In particular, if someone is anxious about "X," they are encouraged to try to *maximize* "X"—a sort of application of the Law of Similars. One example that Frankl mentions in his book is the cure of a lifelong and severe stutterer. Frankl encouraged this patient to try as hard as possible to stutter whenever he was in a situation that would normally trigger stuttering—and it worked! Eventually, he was relieved of his stuttering permanently. Just as in homeopathy, a dose of similar energy served to inform this patient's body/mind of an ingrained pattern and break free.

Finally, another future-oriented meaning-based approach is the use of *positive visualization* to create an intended result. Consider the phenomenon mentioned in Chapter 16—that just by imagining you are exercising, you can strengthen the muscles in your Physical Body. Athletes often use this kind of visualization as part of their training.

But even more can be accomplished if the powerful Causal Body is called into play. As I will discuss in the next chapter, if the Mental Body can formulate the image of a desired result, and if it can also engage both the Astral Body and the Causal Body to assist it, amazing forms of manifestation, creation, and healing can occur.

CHAPTER 18

꒓

WE ARE CREATORS

We have now reached what some people call the High Self—the mysterious and wise Causal Body. This part of us is our connection to the universal creative source—God, Great Spirit, The Force, all that is. The Bible states that we are each created in God's image. Because of this, we have inherent potential for great creative power. But even if you aren't wedded to a spiritual tradition or believe in God, you might still be able to acknowledge that there must be some energetic force that creates everything we experience, and that each of us is a fragment and manifestation of that force. If so, we may also be imbued with at least some of that same creative power.

In general, we aren't aware of our Causal Body most of the time. It is much easier to get in touch with our Astral and Mental bodies—our inner feelings and thoughts. Nevertheless, our Causal Body is always there. The easiest way to make contact is through meditation. By stilling your sensations, feelings, and thoughts, the wisdom and the power of the Causal Body can break through. It can also make itself known at random times—when you are taking a shower, sitting in a quiet forest glen, or in answer to a prayer for guidance. That "still small voice" within you is also mentioned in the Bible. Christians call it "the Christ within" or the Holy Spirit. In Judaism and Hinduism, it is the "I AM." In fact, in the Bible, God's self-description is in a similar form: "I AM THAT I AM"—

although a more accurate translation is: "I WILL BE WHAT I WILL BE," once again emphasizing God's creative power. Your Causal Body, the godly part of you, has great vision and creative power.

In my previous book, *Active Consciousness,*[1] I laid out a grand theory of how the ability to create operates and how we can access it. It goes something like this. At each point in time, each of us is at a gateway to an infinite number of possible futures. Our Causal Body is the part of us that possesses a higher-dimensional power to see those possibilities, as well as the ability to mold the future and guide us along a particular desired pathway forward. In essence, it can influence our possible futures, changing the probability that certain ones actually occur. Amazingly, quantum physics gets closer and closer each day to verifying this idea. There is even some evidence that we can influence and alter the past too.[2] Could it be possible that when we visualize a past traumatic event and imagine it turning out differently, we are not only assuaging our Astral Body and its memories, but also changing those past events?

So how do we enlist this inner power to create the future we desire? And how can we use it to heal ourselves? That is a subject of study and experimentation for many people today and, as it turns out, has been a critical component of esoteric systems of thought for thousands of years. Somehow, this information keeps popping up in a way that is comprehensible and relevant to each time and place. Since we are all human beings with Physical, Etheric, Astral, Mental, and Causal Bodies, perhaps that isn't so surprising. In the past, this perennial wisdom was usually kept secret or was actively suppressed. Today, more and more people are tapping into it and trying to use it to influence their lives.

THE LAW OF ATTRACTION

A common phrase used today for understanding and using the creative power of the Causal Body is "The Law of Attraction." In simple terms, this law states that *what we believe, talk about, and focus on tends to manifest as outer experience.* Those who espouse this concept tend to view the law as a fundamental operating principle of the universe, just like gravity or other physical forces. It's simply the way the world works. Just like gravity, our beliefs and thoughts—whether conscious or unconscious, positive or negative—attract and thereby create our experienced reality.

Can you see how the Law of Attraction is related to synchronicity? Indeed, it may be what *causes* synchronicities. Or perhaps, it is synchronicities that enable the Law of Attraction to operate. For example, if we create a negative field of meaning around us by constantly focusing on something negative or talking about it all of the time, we may actually be *attracting* it to us by creating a negatively-charged synchronicity. In fact, people who always complain about money, relationships, or work woes often *do* lead lives that are plagued by such problems. *But what is cause and what is effect?* Perhaps their habit of negativity is actually enabling these experiences to synchronistically occur. If so, altering their emotional habits could actually change their lives for the better.

Of course, if the Law of Attraction operates on an individual level, it is likely even more powerful on the collective level. Just think about how so much of today's media foments our collective fears about politics, health, conflict, and more. This may actually be a key force that is bringing these fears into fruition! What would happen if the media focused on positive news instead?

That's not to say we should do nothing about the world's injustices and other problems. But productive action is rarely what the media focuses on. Instead, it takes advantage of the addictive power of fear and anger to whip people up into an unproductive—indeed *counter-productive*—frenzy. An alternative would be to reveal and describe the world's problems in more neutral terms, and then focus media excitement on the positive solutions and approaches that people are already engaging in. This would instill hope, provide an incentive for participation, and create a vision of a better future—a vision that if we all engaged in, would increase the probability that it actually occurs.

Along the same lines, what if fictional television shows weren't so often focused on horrific apocalyptic futures and crime, but instead, depicted a world of peace and prosperity? One reason for the enduring appeal of the television show *Star Trek* is that it envisions an Earth in which humanity has gotten its act together and has created a peaceful planet. The show has always inspired hope, despite off-world problems within the Star Trek universe. I'm sure that the scriptwriters who depict horrible near-term futures for Earth may actually have good intentions—perhaps, to alert and activate people to ensure that such futures don't occur. But what if they are actually accomplishing quite the opposite—creating mass visualizations that help bring apocalypses into being?

The bottom line is that the Law of Attraction is a neutral law. We can use it to manifest good or bad. Ideally, it is used for good. And one way to do so is to call upon the Causal Body. Yes, our Astral Body can be misguided and thereby attract negative life experiences with its misguided beliefs and thoughts. Similarly, our Mental Body can be used to formulate and execute negative thoughts and plans too. But if we can heal these parts of ourselves and enlist the wisdom and even greater creative power of our Causal Body, we can use the very same Law of Attraction to create a happier and healthier future instead.

MANIFESTATION/CREATION METHODS BASED ON THE LAW OF ATTRACTION

Workshops about the Law of Attraction have become more commonplace over the past few decades. Even popular teachers and celebrities like Oprah Winfrey and Deepak Chopra talk about it. Indeed, the phrase "Law of Attraction" seems to have become part of the vernacular, at least for a segment of the population. But the idea that we attract what we believe and focus on isn't really new. In this section, I'll talk about writings that touch upon this concept, starting from today and going back in time.

The many writers and teachers who now talk about the Law of Attraction include Esther Hicks (who channels the Abraham teachings),[3] Tosha Silver,[4] Oprah Winfrey,[5] Deepak Chopra,[6] me (in my book *Active Consciousness*),[1] Hale Dwoskin,[7] Joe Dispenza,[8] Wayne Dyer,[9] Louise Hay,[10] Rhonda Byrne (who created the popular movie *The Secret*),[11] and many others. All of these authors describe basically the same technique, albeit with some differences. The Ha Ritual of Huna described in Chapter 9 is another variation on this theme.

Despite the fact that the Law of Attraction may seem like a new idea to most of us, it has been around, in one form or another, for a long time. Back in the 1960s, for example, we had the channeled teachings of Seth that came through Jane Roberts and were recorded in a series of books.[12] Another work that supposedly channels the words of Jesus, *A Course in Miracles*, came forth in the 1970s.[13] These and other channeled teachings of that time were essentially descriptions of the Law of Attraction. I myself was greatly influenced by the writings of Sanaya Roman who channeled an entity called Orin.[14]

Moving back to the mid-1900s, the Law of Attraction underlies the very popular "power of positive thinking" principles of that period, though it tended to be targeted toward business goals. Authors of that genre included Dale Carnegie[15] and Napoleon Hill.[16] Their books were carriers of wisdom promulgated by the *New Thought* movement, which became extremely popular in the early 1900s, especially during the Depression. Among the many popular authors of that time were Neville Goddard (one of my favorites),[17] Florence Scovel Shinn (check out her book *The Game of Life and How to Play It*),[18] James Allen,[19] Norman Vincent Peale,[20] Thomas Troward,[21] and Ernest Holmes, author of *Science of Mind*[22] and founder of a religious movement called Spiritual Science. Today, Spiritual Science is taught at churches called Centers for Spiritual Living,[23] which have inspired many of today's authors, including Louise Hay.

Interestingly, the founder of another spiritual movement, Huna, also began his work during the heyday of the New Thought movement. During his travels to Hawaii in the early 1900s, Max Freedom Long recognized that New Thought principles aligned with the teachings of the Hawaiian shamans he studied with. He combined this information to create the system he called Huna.[24] It is therefore not surprising that the Ha Ritual reflects the Law of Attraction. Many (if not most) of the New Thought teachers also believed that its principles were hidden in the words of great religious figures, especially Jesus.[21] They often quoted biblical texts in their writings to illustrate the fact that New Thought is truly not new at all.

Next, let's not forget that psychiatrist Carl Jung, who first coined the term "synchronicity" in the 1900s, did so during the same time period.[25] Jung's work definitely reflected ideas that were popular in the late 1800s and early 1900s. Another important teacher and philosopher of that period, who was in alignment with the same spiritual principles, was Rudolf Steiner.[26] Steiner was a prolific thinker and developed anthroposophical medicine (partially inspired by homeopathy), Waldorf schools, a movement system called eurythmy, and biodynamic agriculture. Like Barbara Brennan, Steiner was a spiritual adept who could "see" the energy bodies, which he described in his writings. I discuss many of his revelations at length in *Active Consciousness*.

Another significant figure of that period was mystic G.I. Gurdjieff, who traveled and taught throughout the Middle East and Russia. He too stressed the many layers of our being and the critical difference between operating from our almost mechanical physical self versus being guided by our deeper Causal Self. Gurdjieff's teachings were detailed in the book *In Search of the Miraculous*, written by his follower P.D. Ouspensky.[27] I discuss this information at length in *Active Consciousness*, along with my own theory about the higher-dimensional nature of the Astral, Mental, and Causal bodies.

Going back even further to the mid-1800s, we had the *transcendentalist* movement and writers like Ralph Waldo Emerson[28] and Henry David Thoreau,[29] both of whom inspired many in the New Thought movement. Adherents of transcendentalism valued independent spirituality, intuition, and personal awareness over the teachings of conventional religious institutions. Inherent to the philosophy was the assumption that we are all spiritual beings. Transcendentalists also acknowledged the deep interconnectivity between humanity and nature.

Of course, it's not surprising that those in the transcendentalist and New Thought movements were also deeply influenced by teachings from India. One practice in Yogic tradition, *sankalpa*, focuses on impressing positive intentions upon the subconscious mind (the Astral Body), especially while falling asleep—a practice also stressed by New Thought writer Neville Goddard. Given that imminent sleep is the point at which the Astral, Mental, and Causal bodies detach and operate within the astral or higher realms, it is really the perfect time to ask these parts of ourselves to explore future possibilities and to help bring intentions and desires into manifestation.

Another related religious movement that appeared in the mid-1800s was North American Spiritualism,[30] a Christian sect focused on contact with the astral realm and on developing and scientifically testing psychic abilities like mediumship (communication with the dead). The Spiritualist movement is still alive and well today and operates many churches around the world. Another movement born at the same time was Christian Science, founded by Mary Baker Eddy,[31] which focuses on the power of belief to heal the body.

Let's go back even further now into the 1700s. Here we can find the teachings of Emanuel Swedenborg.[32] Swedenborg was an esteemed Swedish scientist who experienced a profound spiritual awakening at age 53. His newly developed psychic powers were considered to be so accurate that Europe's royal families called upon him for advice. After his awakening, Swedenborg wrote numerous books about his insights, which later became the basis for the Swedenborgian church. Among the teachings of this church is the principle of *correspondence*, in which physical objects and events are reflections of principles and ideas in the higher realms of our being. Sounds a bit like the Law of Similars, synchronicity, and the Law of Attraction, doesn't it? Interestingly, many of the homeopaths of the 1800s were Swedenborgians.

But that's not where it ends. Ideas about our true identity as complete human beings go back even further in time and appear in every culture. I have given you just a smattering of examples from European and American history. But the truth is, these concepts go back thousands of years and likely cross-fertilized one another. For example, many people believe that Jesus traveled to India during his "lost years" (ages 12-29) and was influenced by Buddhist teachings there. Many New Thought writers believe that Jesus was simply trying to teach his followers that *everyone* is a Son of God and therefore has the ability to perform healings and other miracles. That is certainly the message of the channeled *A Course in Miracles*.[13] The key idea is that if we are all created in God's image, then we all have the ability to create and manifest with the aid of our higher energy bodies.

Long before the life of Jesus, of course, Jews developed the principle of monotheism—the idea that there is only one creator and that each of us is created in God's image. Some have even posited that the unpronounced name of God in the Bible—Y H V H—is a code or formula for our ability to create. Truthfully, though, this law appears in some form in every religion, including Judaism, Zoroastrianism (which originated at about the same time as Judaism), Buddhism, Hinduism, and later Christianity and Islam. Since we are all humans with Physical, Etheric, Astral, Mental, and Causal Bodies, we naturally keep rediscovering it.

PROBLEMS IN THE CAUSAL BODY

What does it mean to have problems within the Causal Body? In my view, most suspected issues are likely not within the Causal Body itself, but rather, with our *access* to it. In other words, problems rooted within our Physical, Etheric, Astral, and Mental Bodies may be blocking access to this inherently wise and powerful part of us. As a result, we can't line up with it; we can't get in sync with its healing power.

If you are having trouble accessing the wisdom of your Causal Body in meditation or when trying to manifest, I believe that the first place to look for answers is either in your Astral or your Mental Body. For example, if you have been unsuccessful in manifesting something, it may be that your Astral Body doesn't want to create it, is afraid of creating it, or wants to keep things the way they are. Alternatively, your Mental Body may not have formulated your desires clearly enough or doesn't have the focus, discipline, and will to truly set it in motion. Another impediment may be that you are trying to *force* something to happen (usually because of anxiety or fear) rather than trusting in the process and allowing it to unfold—letting things just flow. That's why most manifestation practices stress the need to clear blocks within the Astral and Mental Bodies first. Once you do, your call for aid from your Causal Body can be much more effective.

But there is one other possibility. Perhaps, beyond all understanding, your Causal Body may not want something to occur, or it wants you to experience something difficult for a specific reason. For example, perhaps it created a disease or crisis to enable your growth and development. Or perhaps a planned trip is cancelled because it would have resulted in a deadly accident. Sometimes, only hindsight provides the clearest view, though meditation and contact with your higher energy bodies can also provide answers. The point is, life is mysterious and all we can do is our best with the tools we have. And there are many tools available.

SIGNS AND CAUTIONS FOR THE CAUSAL REALM

As I've said, problems involving the Causal Body are usually problems with accessing or establishing contact with it. One sign of this phenomenon is a feeling of disconnection from your spirit and an inability to trust in higher power or flow. There may also be a nagging sense of "Who am I?" This occurs because, without a connection to the inner core of your being, you feel like an empty shell that is vulnerable to negative emotions like greed, anger, fear, and depression. And because the Law of Attraction is always in operation regardless of your state, it will tend to bring exactly what you *don't* want into physical form.

Remember, too, that if you are seeking help in accessing the causal realm, you must trust your *own* instincts and not simply relegate your power to some guru or practitioner. While there are some enlightened and wise people out there, many self-styled gurus are actually playing out their own issues and manipulating their followers. Personally, I've always been wary of this phenomenon and prefer to learn from a variety of teachers. I then combine the knowledge I gain into a form that works for me.

CAUSALLY-BASED THERAPIES

I often hear about teachers giving seminars, writing books and blogs, and giving lectures about the power of intention, the Law of Attraction, and how to harness our amazing human power to create and manifest the things we want in life.   In this section, I'll focus on some of this information and try to put it into a more general framework that, hopefully, will make it easier to understand.

Let me begin by saying that my book *Active Consciousness*[1] presents my own take on the manifestation process. I also try to explain *why* it takes the form it does, in terms of a theory that I present—about how we are higher-dimensional creatures carving a path through the innumerable possibilities existing in higher dimensional space. If you're interested in learning more about this idea as well as a variety of esoteric teachings, studies of psychic phenomena, and a series of lessons on meditation, I highly recommend you read *Active Consciousness*.

The Basic Manifestation/Creation Process

The first step when engaging in any kind of work with the Causal Body is to enter into a meditative state. If you have never meditated before, I recommend buying a book on meditation, taking a course, or joining a meditation group. Such resources can be found almost anywhere these days. Naturally, there are many methods of meditation, each with it own emphasis. Some are religious in nature, others are not. The fundamental idea is to sit, relax, and clear the mind. Some meditation methods focus on breathing techniques, others on reciting a mantra or repetitive statement within the mind, and others simply ask you to focus on body sensations, including sounds in the environment. The short meditation course presented in *Active Consciousness* utilizes the body-sensation method.

If you would like to seek out more personalized help, practitioners like shamans are adept at helping their clients enter into a meditative state and making contact with their Causal Body. Practitioners affiliated with spiritual centers (like the Centers for Spiritual Living) can also help people engage with manifestation and creation for healing purposes. But much can also be accomplished on your own.

Once you have some meditation practice under your belt, you can try out the four-step manifestation/creation process I describe in *Active Consciousness*, which is summarized below. All other methods that I've learned about can be viewed as embellishments on this basic theme. Before you engage with this process, use your powerful Mental Body to create a specific goal statement or intention and write it down. When you do, make sure it has a positive form, as if it were already true. For example, instead of writing "I want to cure my asthma," you could write something like "I always breathe freely and easily." Now you can begin.

1. **NOW+.** Enter into a meditative state. Once you feel you are in the Now moment and have cleared your mind of past memories and future worries, enhance this state with a feeling of gratitude, compassion, and joy. I call this state of being *Now+*. One way to achieve it is to put a slight smile on your face.

2. **PURE GOAL.** Bring your intention into consciousness. Use your powerful Mental Body to focus on it completely, with absolute conviction that it is true right now. Do not try to visualize *how* it will come into being. Instead, use visualization and imagination to bring yourself into a state in which your intention is already fulfilled. Truly *be* in your goal state, without any doubt. Feel it in your body, emotions, and mind. Try to imagine it in a detailed way.

3. **LET GO.** Now come out of the meditative state and leave your intention in the capable hands of your Causal Body. It can also be helpful to say a statement that formally releases the intention and demonstrates your trust in the fact that it will appear. Science of Mind communities utilize the statement "And So It Is." Now, as you go through your days, continue to trust that your intention will manifest. Be alert for feelings of doubt or other negative thoughts about the outcome. If doubts do come up, replace them

with a feeling of confidence and certainty, perhaps by saying your positive intention statement out loud.

4. **CHOOSE JOY.** In general, an intended goal doesn't simply show up on your doorstep. (Though such things have been known to happen!) Instead, you must continue to participate in life, making choices along the way. Be aware that you should try not to have any fixed idea about how your goal will manifest itself. But it can be helpful to consult your Causal Body whenever you do need to make a decision that you are uncertain about. Enter into a light meditative state and bring your choice into awareness. Test out the options in your mind. Choose the option that creates a light feeling of happiness and joy within you, in contrast to one that evokes a more negative feeling. Try to make sure that these sensations are emanating from your wise Causal Body, not your fearful Astral Body. Although the joyful choice may not be the "logical" one, try to follow it anyway.

EMBELLISHMENTS ON THE THEME

I will now present a few other manifestation methods in terms of this basic process. Note that each one represents a significant field of study in its own right. Choose the method that feels best for you.

Huna

I have already described the Ha ritual of Huna in Chapter 9. In contrast to some manifestation methods, Huna recognizes the innate independence and role of each of our physical and energy bodies and explicitly asks them to engage in the process. The Mental Body is enlisted first to provide focus and a description of the intended goal in a useful form. After breathing exercises performed by the Physical Body, the Etheric Body is asked to build up and provide sufficient energy or mana so that the intention can be transmitted by the Astral Body up to the Causal Body.

Indeed, Huna recognizes that it is the Astral Body that is truly the lynchpin of the Ha ritual. That is why physical actions like lighting candles and setting up a written intention statement are involved in the process, all of which make a significant impression upon the Astral Body. Not only is this part of you asked to cooperate and transmit the intention up through the central channel to the Causal Body, but Huna also stresses that an effort must be made in advance to clear conscious and subconscious emotional obstacles in order to guarantee success.

The Teachings of Neville Goddard

Neville Goddard[17] is one of my favorite New Thought teachers. As was true of Huna's developer Max Freedom Long, Goddard liked to write about how biblical and other holy texts subtly convey the idea that our thoughts and beliefs create our reality. I find his books to be especially powerful because they include true stories of manifestation success. He also diverges from some New Thought teachers by placing greater emphasis on how a goal intention is stated and visualized. In particular, he stressed that it is important to focus on a goal state that is a *consequence* of what is intended rather than the primary intention itself.

For example, suppose that you would like to be healed of an ailment. Rather than having a goal like "I am free of asthma" or "I always breathe freely," he suggested visualizing what you would do if you *already had* what you wanted. In the case of asthma, for instance, you might visualize running or doing some other activity easily. I can think of at least two reasons why this approach may be most successful. One is that focusing directly on what you want can sometimes create a sense of separation from it. For example, if you use "I always breathe freely," you may simultaneously become more aware of the fact that you currently *aren't* breathing freely. A second reason for focusing on a goal's consequence is that it is often easier to believe in and imagine. When a visualized scenario can easily be played out in the imagination, it is then much more effective at achieving the PURE GOAL state.

As another illustration, suppose that you would like to have more money. Instead of visualizing "I have a million dollars," imagine engaging in an activity that would be enabled if you had more money— perhaps taking a luxurious vacation, paying for a child to attend an expensive university, or handing an enormous donation check to your favorite charity.

Goddard also emphasized that faith and belief in your visualization is key. He suggested repeating the visualization exercise daily, especially at night in bed before sleep. I've experimented with Goddard's technique on a few relatively simple tasks and met with some surprising successes.

The Teachings of Joe Dispenza

Chiropractor Joe Dispenza, well-known for his work on how to create healing, has become a popular author and teacher in recent years. Dispenza suffered a catastrophic spinal injury when he was a young man. Faced with possible paralysis or undergoing a surgery that would likely leave him in pain for the rest of his life, he made an unusual choice. He decided to try and heal himself. Confined to bed for months, he spent that time visualizing the complete healing of his spine—and he succeeded!

One thing I love about Dispenza's books is that he explains how self-healing might work from the standpoint of current medical understanding—that is, how solely using the mind and emotions *could* translate into known physical healing mechanisms, even if most doctors think it to be impossible. I highly recommend one of his most popular books, *You Are the Placebo*.[8] The title is obviously a delightful jab at quackbusters who use the term "placebo" derisively to negate the miraculous power of self-healing. (I did much the same with the title of my first book, *Impossible Cure: The Promise of Homeopathy*.)

Dispenza's healing technique is based on an extended meditative process in which the meditator reaches an extremely deep state of joy and expansion before visualizing the goal state. In other words, his process places a special emphasis on creating what I would call a supercharged version of NOW+. Maybe it should be called NOW++! Whenever I engage in one of his meditations, I really do have an intensely positive experience.

Dispenza's teachings also emphasize that heightened positive emotions are the key to changing the brain and body, thereby enabling new habits of thought and feeling to take root. I particularly like one analogy he utilizes. Imagine that your current beliefs, habits, and body are like deep ruts in a hard sand beach. Your life will continue along these ruts by default, and they will feel most comfortable and familiar to you. Trying to veer away from them, however, will feel "wrong" or unpleasant. However, if you engage in highly positive emotions while in a meditative state, it's like washing away the ruts with a super charged wave. This allows a new pattern to be established in the sand. In his large group seminars, Dispenza has measured the brain waves and other physiological and emotional measurements of participants and scientifically established the veracity of his theory and the effectiveness of his method. Using it, your brain and body literally *are* freed to sync up with a new state of being.

CLEARING OBSTACLES

As should be obvious by now, unproductive emotions and outdated or erroneous beliefs can be your greatest obstacles to creating and manifesting. That is why so many practitioners and teachers emphasize working with your Astral Body first. In addition to all of the techniques described in Chapter 16, here are some more ideas to consider.

The Teachings of Abraham Hicks

The teachings of the entity Abraham, channeled by Esther Hicks (and therefore sometimes called "Abraham Hicks"), include many exercises that can help you to replace negative thoughts and emotions with more positive ones. One strategy is to compare two thoughts by asking "Which thought feels better?" Another is to gradually move up a scale of twenty-two emotional states that range from "Fear-Grief-Depression-Despair-Powerlessness" at the bottom to "Joy-Knowledge-Empowerment-Freedom-Love-Appreciation" at the top. I've printed out this emotional scale and often look at it to identify where my feelings are on any particular day. Then I try to bump myself up at least one notch—for example, from "Contentment" to "Hopefulness."

The Abraham Hicks teachings also include a lot of information related to Steps 3 and 4 of the basic manifestation process described earlier: LET GO and CHOOSE JOY. For example, they suggest telling yourself that once you have engaged with your intention, you must leave it up to the "Universal Manager" to work things out for you. This may sound a bit silly, but that kind of language and thinking can be helpful. Another idea they stress is to trust what they call your "inner guidance system." This is their way of describing your emotional reactions to choices you must make, knowing that a feeling of internal joy and contentment usually indicates the correct choice and that you are on the right track. Esther Hicks has published several books; an excellent one is *The Amazing Power of Deliberate Intent*.[2]

The Science of Mind

Practitioners of Ernest Holmes' Science of Mind[22] utilize a variety of methods for what he called "spiritual mind treatment"—that is, ways to transform unproductive beliefs into more positive and productive ones. For example, they emphasize that you should become alert to the words you habitually use, many of which reinforce negative states. Constantly complaining, for example, is a sure recipe for perpetuating the things you are complaining about. By training yourself to notice what you say and change your words to be more positive, you actively influence your obedient Astral Body. Don't forget, it's always listening!

A lot of Holmes' teachings also emphasize sustained forms of education. By frequently engaging in Science of Mind reading, lectures, and videos, followers of these teachings better enable their Astral and Mental Bodies to buy into the idea that changing one's life experience really *is* possible. Repetition also cultivates a deeper faith in truly LETTING GO.

Some More Thoughts on Letting Go

The ability to let go is really about trust. I often use the phrase "Trust in Great Spirit." In fact, I say it so much that my son Max made me a little hand-drawn poster with those words on it! Unfortunately, cultivating trust in today's world can be a hard thing to do. The media is constantly bombarding us and encouraging us to be fearful, angry, and *dis*trustful of others. As a result, letting go can be difficult.

Of course, things won't always go your way, even if you do succeed in letting go. But if you've lived enough years, you probably know that hard times usually do have a silver lining, and that the lessons you end up learning can often change your life for the better. Besides, even when death comes knocking on your door, trusting in Great Spirit's ultimate plan can be helpful.

Honestly, I'm not a person who is naturally endowed with equanimity. But in recent years, I've improved quite a bit. For me, Sedona releases and reading certain books have been the most helpful way to make progress with the "trust and let go" piece of life. When things get me down and I need to boost my trust quotient, I do a Sedona release (one of my favorites is "Opening to the River of Life," which I listened to every night during our voyage across America) or I reread a helpful book. Two books that I have found to be particularly useful are: *The Trust Frequency* by Andrew Cameron Bailey and Connie Baxter Marlow[33] and *The Surrender Experiment* by Michael Singer.[34]

Finally, I try to remember Lao-Tzu's famous maxim, *"By letting it go, it all gets done. The world is won by those who let it go. But when you try and try, the world is beyond the winning."* In other words, stop pushing. Trust in Great Spirit and your own inner wisdom and agency. Let it flow. These are truly the keys to living in synchrony.

CHAPTER 19

᠀

YOU ARE NOT ALONE

W e've now considered the many different layers of our complete
Selves, how they affect us, and how they can be healed from an
individual perspective. But we are not isolated beings. We may feel like
we are, as we struggle with our personal aches, pains, and sorrows. But in
truth, each of us is swimming in vast milieus operating at every level,
from physical to causal. And not only does everything within these
collective milieus affect us, but we affect them too. Thus, if our goal is to
live in synchrony, we must learn to not only align within ourselves and
tune into our own environment, but to also consider our role within it.

In this chapter I'll consider a variety of healing modalities that can
help us collectively. Because they range from the physical to the causal in
their application, I'll organize my presentation accordingly. In the next
and final chapter, I'll conclude with a few more thoughts about our
unified existence, along with a recap of lessons learned.

BEING PART OF A COLLECTIVE

Whether we like it or not, whether we believe it or not, and whether
we're aware of it or not, what's going on around us affects us in
profound ways—both positively and negatively. Certainly we can all
agree that if someone spews toxins into the air, water, or soil, your health

will be affected. And if someone drives chaotically on the road without paying attention to traffic signals, others will experience the consequences. Science is also beginning to recognize that electromagnetic radiation, such as that emanating from cell phones and Wi-Fi, is affecting us in unseen ways, causing syndromes that range from insomnia to diabetes, heart disease, cancer, and neurological disorders. And why shouldn't this be so? We are energy beings after all. Luckily, a healthy physical environment, well-regulated traffic, and a natural energy environment can yield positive healing effects. That's why folks put so much effort into cleaning things up in those spheres.

Going up another level to the astral realm, we all know what it's like to spend a lot of time in a toxic emotional atmosphere. If chronic anger, violence, and fear are constantly swirling all around us, these emotions tend to seep into our beings whether we are conscious of it or not. Children who grow up in emotionally toxic households can be affected for life and, in fact, these effects can be inherited too. For example, studies have shown that the traumas experienced by Holocaust survivors created emotional and physiological effects that appear not only in their children, but in their grandchildren too. Consider then, how the collective traumas of our ancestors may be affecting us.

Do you doubt that this is possible? As described in Chapter 3, research conducted by Dean Radin and Roger Nelson demonstrated that even *machines* can pick up on collective emotional states.[1] In 1997, they placed random event generators at fifty locations all around the world and ran them continuously to see if they could be affected by significant world events. The results were astounding. Over the next ten years, Radin and Nelson studied the machines' reactions to 205 major world events and discovered that they did indeed respond to those that were intense on a global level—especially tragic events. The most striking effects occurred on 9/11, which caused the largest daily average correlation between the machines' outputs. Even more amazing, this correlation began a few hours *before* the twin towers were hit. Was this an instance of collective precognition? And if mechanical devices can pick up on our collective emotional energy, how much more deeply do we humans? After all, we evolved to pick up on such things.

Unfortunately, chronic widespread anger and fear have become even more prevalent in recent years. Thanks to the instantaneous media stew that envelops us, we may all be experiencing a collective form of PTSD (post traumatic stress disorder). Is that why depression and anxiety are so prevalent today, even among children? And remember: these effects aren't just emotional; they can be physical too.

Of course, there were collective emotional traumas in the past too, and they also likely caused collective physical disease. For instance, you might think that the Spanish flu epidemic, which killed so many people after World War I, was simply a matter of physical pathogens being spread around by soldiers returning home from the war. But what if the epidemic was actually caused, or at least exacerbated, by an *emotional* trauma that affected so many people at that time?

The homeopathic remedy that was extremely successful in treating the Spanish flu (with a death rate of 1-3% versus a death rate of 30% among conventional doctors) was *Gelsemium*. This remedy remains one of the most important flu remedies to this day. On an emotional level, Gelsemium's symptoms match a wartime and post-war emotional state very well: anxiety and fearful anticipation with trembling, a desire to be held, wanting to be quiet and undisturbed, and weeping. Is it so surprising that soldiers and their families who experienced these emotional symptoms became susceptible to a flu virus that could be cured by *Gelsemium*? What is cause and what is effect? These are important questions to ask today, as the world becomes enveloped in a growing number of pandemics and armed conflicts.

In summary, individual and collective illness caused by group-level phenomena is real. That is why group-level healing methods can be so effective. Indigenous societies all over the world have always known this. When humanity was composed of small tribes, the collective tribal state of consciousness was an important consideration when it came to healing. When a member of a tribe or family was ill, the first place healers looked for answers was the larger unit in which that person lived—that is, what was going on in their physical and emotional environment. Rituals were then utilized to purify these collective physical, energetic, emotional, and mental energies. The primacy we now give to individual health and wellness is a relatively recent phenomenon.

Another thing that was recognized by indigenous societies was the impact of the wider physical environment and its energies, especially that of nearby animal populations. Today, we may laugh at the notion that the wrath of a buffalo herd or of a disturbed lake or forest spirit could affect us humans. But at the deepest levels of our being, who can say this is not true? The animals, the water, the trees and plants, the mountains, the atmosphere—they all have consciousness too. And this consciousness *does* affect us.

Planet Earth is suffering. Species are going extinct. Pollution is rampant. Is this only being caused by humanity's careless use of resources? Is it simply due to reckless dumping of toxins into our air, soil, and water? Or do things go much deeper? Are collective toxic energies from humanity at the etheric, astral, and mental levels wreaking havoc upon the planet itself? Of course, it likely goes in the other direction too. Planetary weather events like volcanic eruptions, solar flares, earthquakes, and tsunamis affect us individually and collectively at every level. Again, what is cause and what is effect?

Consider the fact that family units are increasingly breaking down and cultural structures are being radically altered. Negative emotions have become inflamed, mental fog is commonplace even among the young, and escapism into drugs, overconsumption, and other diversions has become the norm. So many of us are swamped by feelings of disconnection and ennui, made worse by the materialistic belief that we are all just biological machines disconnected from our environment and each other. Indeed, some of us are beginning to wake up to the possibility that forces that would like to use this dysfunction to enact global forms of power and control are helping to orchestrate this state of affairs.

Luckily, there is a solution that few have yet considered, and if you've read this far, you may be able to guess what it is. The fact is, *we are not disconnected biological machines*. We are powerful energy beings— even more powerful if we act together. Naturally, we need to stop engaging in obviously harmful physical and etheric pollution. But healing at higher levels of our being could have an even more potent impact. What if we heal at a global emotional level, starting with our families and working our way up to communities, cities, regions, and countries? What if we clear our collective minds and our sense of purpose returns? What if we ignite our causal power and intentionally create healing for the entire planet? I will discuss this further in Chapter 20. For now, let's look at various forms of collective healing that are currently available, starting at the physical level and working our way upward.

COLLECTIVE HEALING AT THE PHYSICAL LEVEL

If we want to be healthy physically, we must live in a healthy physical environment, eat healthy food, drink healthy water, and act in a healthy way. But going at it alone, each of us trying to clean up our own act, isn't cutting it anymore. The difficulties have become too overwhelming. Many of us feel like Sisyphus, pushing the boulder of our own personal health uphill against the gravity of an environment that keeps pushing us down. What can be done?

One step that most developed societies have taken is cleaning up and protecting the water supply and establishing a good sanitation infrastructure. In fact, many of the epidemics of the 1800s and early 1900s (including polio) were not actually alleviated by vaccination programs but, instead, by improved sanitation and water systems that were built at around the same time. In regions around the world where this has not been true, acute epidemic diseases are still a major problem.

Another important requirement for collective health is improving the physical structures in which we live. That's why building codes have been developed to ensure that we live in safe dwellings. Unfortunately, however, new problems inevitably arise. Most of us know now about the danger of molds. Less acknowledged is the toxic off-gassing of modern building materials, furnishings, carpets, cleaning supplies, and even clothing. Ideally, safer materials will eventually become affordable to all, rather than being a solution available only to the wealthy. And let's not forget the dangers of water fluoridation that are only now becoming recognized and admitted by authorities in power. It's unfathomable that we've allowed industries to dump their fluoride by-products (along with other toxins) into our water and air under the guise that they are innocuous or "helpful" in some way.

Perhaps assuring clean air and water will always be a struggle. But the fact is, all of us, rich and poor, need to breathe our collective air and drink our shared water. So, there is no choice but to work collectively to prevent industries from polluting these precious resources, and in particular, from dumping toxins into poorer communities that have less power to protect themselves.

Next comes the food we eat. We must admit to ourselves that foods laced with pesticides (or in some cases, GMO foods that have pesticides genetically embedded within them) aren't healthy for anyone. What are we thinking, allowing our food supply and soil to become contaminated with these toxins? Monoculture practices and pesticides have now depleted our soils drastically, and foods aren't as nutritious as they were just 50 years ago. Bee populations have become endangered, threatening the viability of growing many foods.

Yes, we can each try to buy healthier foods as individuals, but once again, general awareness of the problem is lacking and affordability tends to confine this option to the wealthy. We must work collectively to protect the food supply for *everyone*—a battle that, unfortunately, must also be fought against powerful corporate interests. Luckily, regenerative agricultural practices do exist that can help to correct these problems. (Watch the amazing movie "The Biggest Little Farm" to see an example of this.[2]) In fact, regenerative agriculture even has the power to heal our water supplies and air. Win win!

We must also work together to ignite awareness of the true reasons for the obesity epidemic that is threatening our collective health. It isn't that we are eating too much, but rather, that the foods we eat are inherently flawed and unhealthy. If you travel to Europe, you will not see the widespread obesity that has become the norm in the United States and Canada. Why? For one thing, GMOs are banned in many countries there. Second, the companies that make American junk foods are actually forced by European laws to make healthier versions of the exact same products to sell there. The Europeans have done it; why can't North Americans?

And what about the non-food items we willingly dump into our physical bodies? We inject way too many vaccines laced with aluminum and mercury and ingest way too many pills on a daily basis. Our bodies simply can't take it anymore. Even children have become chronically ill. Unfortunately, this has become the new norm. Young parents don't realize that the extent of chronic disease seen in today's children was unheard of fifty years ago. Sadly, even with the benefits of modern allopathy, life expectancy is now going down, at least in the United States.

So what can we do to stop the pharmaceutical steamroller? First, we have to recognize the folly of our reliance on drug-based solutions. Already, the overuse of antibiotics (not just prescribed pills, but also embedded in household products and used prophylactically in farm animals) has led to antibiotic resistant strains of bacteria that are fast becoming a serious collective health threat. Hospitals are no longer safe places in which to get well but, instead, danger zones where patients can easily be exposed to drug resistant infections.

Next, we must collectively insist that advertising and promotion of drugs in the media be forbidden. This phenomenon began in the 1980s. Before that time, suggesting the use of a drug was solely the purview of doctors, not advertisers. Today, we are bombarded by nonstop *nocebos* that scare us into fear and foreboding, courtesy of the pharmaceutical industry, which has bought and controlled our government representatives and the media. In some cases, we are even legally forced into medical compliance—supposedly for "our own good."

As an individual, it's critical that you become aware of all of this and do what you can to dispel its effects upon you. Don't forget, your Astral Body is always listening and has a great influence upon your physical well-being. It is extremely important to actively tell yourself that you will not be influenced by media nocebos. One approach that I use when I hear a nocebo message coming my way is to say out loud: *"I am an infinite being and I am not subject to that. That does not apply to me and I hereby refuse and cancel that information."* In the long run, however, collective efforts to stem this tide are the only real answer.

Finally, let's talk about behavior. Let's do something collectively to improve how we move our Physical Bodies. I remember back in middle school gym class, there was a yearly "posture queen" competition. Not surprisingly, it became the butt of many jokes; *no one* wanted to be posture queen! But what if every elementary school child was taught the Gokhale Method and learned how to properly sit, stand, walk, and sleep at a young age? Lifelong aches and pains could be averted and billions of dollars in health care costs would be saved.

Indeed, what if chairs and car seats were restructured to promote correct posture rather accommodating poor ones? What if physical education classes were focused less on competitive sports and redirected toward exercise and agility? What if all children were taught Yoga, Qi Gong, or other movement therapies that could provide lifelong health benefits? I recall being at a public festival in Rejkjavik, Iceland that included vendors and games for children. Yes, there were junk foods being sold. But the park space was also filled with health-promoting physical games for the children to enjoy. Stilts, climbing structures, balance boards, and other devices that promote strength and agility were scattered all about and the children had lots of fun using them. It was a huge contrast with similar kinds of events in the United States.

In summary, we can do quite a lot collectively on the physical level to create a healthier world for all of us. But there's much to be done at the energetic levels too. Remember: the higher up we go, the more powerful we can be, especially when we work together.

COLLECTIVE HEALING AT THE ETHERIC LEVEL

Have you ever considered the fact that bacteria and viruses have Etheric Bodies too? I've heard one very interesting hypothesis—that bacterial and viral diseases aren't *caused* by germs but rather, by toxic etheric energies that *attract* these germs. In other words, the presence of "harmful" germs is merely a sign that the true source of harm—toxic energies—are present, just as the presence of ants in your house is a sign that a sugary substance has been left out. Clean up the energy (the sugar) and the pests will leave too. And perhaps that's why homeopathic and other etheric approaches to bacterial and viral infections are so successful. Once the correct energy-based remedy heals your Etheric Body, the bacteria and viruses leave the scene and your Physical Body can heal itself.

So how could this play out at a collective level? First, be aware that harmful influences aren't just physical and that you can improve your health by eliminating negative mental, etheric, and astral energies. Doctors in hospitals know this very well. They simply decide that they won't get sick and they usually don't. In other words, they mentally and astrally—and by extension, etherically—block disease energies. You can do this too. When you find yourself in a crowd of coughing and sneezing people, imagine a golden ball of energy protecting you. I've also had some success imagining blue energy cleansing troublesome areas in my body.

Next, remember that the etheric realm is highly affected by electromagnetic energy. Many suspect that autism, Alzheimer's, depression, insomnia, and other problems have been accelerated by electromagnetic frequencies (EMFs) that we are increasingly exposed to every day. These EMFs emerge from cell towers, cell phones, Wi-Fi, cordless phones, smart meters, and more. Just as we need to clean up our food, water, and air, we need to use our collective will to clean up our EMF environment. Yes, you can try to remove these influences from your home as an individual. But ultimately, this toxic energetic soup is becoming inescapable. We need to remove these influences or at least mitigate them with technological solutions that hopefully can be discovered. Biogeometry, perhaps? And remember that young children are especially prone to EMF injury. Parents: be aware!

What about the general etheric "vibe" of a region? Yes, every home has its vibe or gestalt. You can feel it when you walk inside a dwelling. But communities, cities, and even countries have their own unique vibe too—and it may or may not blend well with your own vibration. It's always wise, then, to become aware of how the energies of the community or location in which you live affect you.

Some locations, of course, feel good to almost everyone and that's why we tend to take vacations there. Perhaps it's the etheric energy of the surrounding natural terrain—for example, that which is found in places like Sedona, Arizona or on tropical islands. It's not just their physical beauty that affects us; it's their etheric energy, which includes the energies of plants, animals, water, mountains, and soil.

Sadly, however, even these locations are becoming challenged by overdevelopment, tourism, and pollution. Native cultures know that cutting down certain trees, altering certain land formations, or polluting the soil and water affects things in not just a physical way; it damages the innate etheric energy of a region. In response, they devised healing rituals, prayers, and ceremonies to heal these etheric (as well as astral, mental, and perhaps even causal) energies. They openly apologize to the plants, animals, mountains, water, and air and ask for their cooperation when unnatural development occurs. This kind of wisdom can help all of us.

Finally, many of the healing modalities described in Chapter 15 can be applied collectively. For instance, there have been many successful efforts at using homeopathic remedies to prevent epidemic diseases. One was a leptospirosis epidemic in Cuba that was averted for several years by nationwide dissemination of a homeopathic prophylactic.[3] Another was a meningitis epidemic in Argentina that was stopped in its tracks by mass homeopathic treatment.[4] Similar successful efforts have been used in Africa to avert and treat AIDS and malaria.[5]

The homeopathic approach to epidemics, whether of known or unknown origin, is to collect enough data about patient symptoms to determine the *genus epidemicus*—a small set of remedies that will be useful for most people. Once this set is determined, homeopaths can provide prophylactic doses as well as rapidly and effectively treat affected patients on a large scale. This type of collective homeopathic treatment is particularly powerful because homeopathic remedies are essentially cost-free and easy to disseminate. If only homeopathy were recognized and accepted everywhere! Unfortunately, the pharmaceutical industry has been busy discrediting and blocking access to it for this very reason; it's bad for business.

Remember, too, that homeopathic remedies are essentially vibrations. Collective use of vibration can also be used in other ways. The use of sound as a collective healing technique, for instance, has been growing in popularity in recent years. By attending "sound baths," whole groups of people can be healed by the etheric energies of sound. Similarly, many in India know that some gurus can emanate healing energies that transform everyone in their presence, and that certain ragas (traditional Indian music) have specific healing effects.

What if these kinds of vibrations could be "bottled" and shared everywhere? Some homeopaths have been trying to do just that. They have been experimenting with capturing the energy of remedies as sounds and transmitting them over the internet as audio files. The same could be done with any form of sound. The potential of this kind of healing has only begun to be explored and its impact could be enormous and profound. Personally, I believe that sound will become a leading healing technology of the 21st century.

COLLECTIVE HEALING AT THE ASTRAL LEVEL

Now let's consider collective healing at the emotional astral level. We all know that family and workplace dramas can cause stress in our lives and that emotional stress can cause physical disease. But what is "stress"? Is it just a name for a chemical process that causes inflammation in our bodies? No! It's an actual energetic stressor within our Astral Bodies that can potentially remain with us for a lifetime. It can even be passed down to our descendants. Astral injuries can also be implanted within us in the womb or when we are small babies. They may also be completely unconscious to us.

Of course, such injuries don't only occur on an individual basis. Collective astral wounds can be found in families, countries, and cultures. Family patterns of anger, fear, and guilt can lead to multi-generational tendencies for specific physical and emotional diseases. Work environments can breed emotionally toxic patterns of energy. Religious sects or cults can be infected with contagious paranoia and hatred. Governments can instill collective fear in their populace—even infecting the Astral Body of the country itself—in order to drum up support for wars or other political aims. Fear energies can even create changes in our physical environment.

Consider, for example, how the Astral Body of Germany itself (the country) was affected by what happened during the Holocaust. Some people are aware of this wound and have actively tried to heal it. I can tell you from personal experience that the emotional trauma of the Holocaust definitely affected the Astral Bodies of Jewish people all over the world, not just those who were directly affected. Seventy years later, Jews are still working out this collective trauma, whether they are conscious of it or not. And, of course, it affected the Astral Bodies of the perpetrators and the rest of the German population too. The same goes for collective wounds caused by slavery in America, which still affects the United States today. Thus, collective astral wounds within humanity are very real, universal, and long lasting.

What about the collective power of *nocebos*—negative health messages and apocalyptic scenarios that bombard us daily through every form of media? TV shows, movies, advertisements about illnesses and drugs, social media, government warnings and laws, messaging from insurance companies, conversations with friends and family—all of these can scare our Astral Bodies into unnecessary illnesses. The result is a kind of collective hypnosis. Was it actually a virus that caused your flu? Or was it all those signs in the supermarket and pharmacy telling you to get your flu shot—convincing your Astral Body that it should definitely create the flu for you? Even horoscopes in the media can affect our collective emotional Astral Bodies.

So what can we do?

First, you need to become aware that this is happening. Try to avoid nocebos and tell your emotional Astral Body—preferably out loud—that these negative messages do not apply to you. Be aware of how collective messages of fear, paranoia, and hatred affect you, and actively try to dispel them. Meditation can help too.

There are collective methods of astral healing too. Examples include group family therapy, workshops designed to enable adversaries to talk and listen to one another with compassion (e.g., dialogue efforts aimed at inner city gangs), and real efforts at taking societal actions to heal affected groups. The amazing work of Thomas Hübl[6] on healing collective trauma is particularly significant. Remember that physical actions are extremely important. It's not enough to simply "think" about healing; something must be done in the outer world. It might include reparations for victims of atrocities and the erection of memorial monuments and remembrance museums. Germany has engaged in all of these actions to help heal the wounds of the Holocaust. These efforts are not empty gestures, and they help to heal collective astral wounds for *both* sides—both perpetrators and victims.

Collective healing strategies are also part of a Hawaiian practice called *Ho'oponopono*, which means "to bring about rightness." In recent years, the term has grown in popularity and is associated with four healing phrases: "I love you," "I'm sorry," "Thank you," "Please forgive me." But this formula is a gross simplification of a complex healing process.

As a culture, the native Hawaiians realize that sickness within an individual can be a sign that the Astral Body of an entire family unit needs to be healed. Typically, a shaman or wise elder is brought in to guide the Ho'oponopono process, which follows very specific guidelines. Some families also engage in Ho'oponopono regularly in order to prevent illness from occurring in the first place. A Ho'oponopono ritual might also be invoked when a family member experiences a bad omen or in order to facilitate a birth in a family that has suffered from discord.

The goal of Ho'oponopono, as its meaning suggests, is to set things right and heal energies within the collective. Family members are expected to make every effort to attend, even if it requires traveling great distances. The process takes several hours or even days or weeks and can be extremely emotional and difficult, requiring breaks and "cooling off" periods. It begins with a prayer to bring in the family's guardian spirits so that they can assist in the process. The next steps are as follows: identify the problems; state the transgressions; discussion (which can reveal deeper layers); identify negative entanglements; share feelings; confessions and other agreed-upon restitutions; ceremonial release of problems; cutting off problems energetically; summarizing and reaffirming bonds; and a closing prayer followed by a meal.

Just imagine how this healing method could be applied more widely—in couples, businesses and governments, communities, and in circles of friends. However, Ho'oponopono requires participation and sincerity in order to be truly effective. It also requires participants to acknowledge the importance of collective healing on the emotional astral level.

COLLECTIVE HEALING AT THE MENTAL LEVEL

As the saying goes, "Where there's a will, there's a way." Losing the will to live or to accomplish anything in life is bad enough on an individual level. What does it mean when an entire group of people experiences a wound in their collective Mental Body and loses its will? Many feel that this occurred and affected the entire world during the COVID pandemic. People have also become traumatized by the nature of messaging about climate change.

As many spiritual teachers have stressed, our thoughts and beliefs create our reality. When we constantly focus on hopelessness and negative images of the future, we can literally create these outcomes. Remember, too, what Victor Frankl discovered in the concentration camps: those who gave up all hope died within days. In contrast, those who found a way to visualize survival and something to live for, despite all evidence to the contrary, were able to survive even the most dire circumstances. Wise leaders know this. That's why Franklin Roosevelt gave Americans strength during the Depression and World War II by reminding them that "the only thing to fear is fear itself."

Unfortunately, we are experiencing much the opposite these days. A lot of it is due to various weather catastrophes, economic collapse, war, and pandemic disease. Symptoms of our collective wound include not only emotional symptoms like depression and anxiety, but also a mental loss of will reflected in ennui and addiction to drugs and other activities like eating, shopping, and social media.

Another sign of our collective mental wound is a loss of rationality. Indeed, fear is well known to disable rational thought processes. This can result in not only widespread mental fog, but also the acceptance of behavior and ideas that would have previously been rejected—for example, irrational scapegoating. Power hungry individuals take advantage of this collective state so that they can amass more power and control. And be aware that this can happen on *all* sides of any issue. As Mattias Desmet pointed out in his brilliant book, *The Psychology of Totalitarianism*,[7] this phenomenon can lead to mass psychological states that enable the rise of totalitarianism. It's already happening in the world today, just as was true before World War II. We see it in the growing acceptance of surveillance, digital forms of identification used to control behavior and finances, and ever-increasing censorship.

Of course, collective Mental Body suffering has been around for a long time—perhaps for as long as humanity has been in existence. I came face to face with one example of it in 2014, when my husband Steve and I took our first driving trip together across the United States. Up until that time, I had only experienced the East and West coasts. What an eye opener that trip was! To our dismay, we discovered that many once thriving cities had fallen into ruin. For example, in the capital city of Pierre, South Dakota, beautiful older homes were visibly crumbling from disrepair. The only real activity going on was on the outskirts of town, peppered by motels for interstate travelers, casinos, and "gun and pawn" shops (a common combination we saw throughout our travels). Also ubiquitous were road signs that exhorted people not to take methamphetamine.

The people we met throughout our trip were extremely friendly—indeed, much friendlier than folks on the coasts. But without real employment prospects, hope had drained from these communities. The collective Mental Body wounds were obvious. What they needed was some form of community logotherapy—a way for their region to find purpose and meaning once again. In recent years, this phenomenon is becoming apparent in the big coastal cities too.

Of course, ennui, escapist addiction, and scapegoating aren't unique to the United States. It can be found everywhere. The changes we are all experiencing these days are world-wide. No wonder many people live in denial or at least try to avoid thinking about it. The internet and other media have also contributed to these collective Mental Body wounds, serving as potent and addictive lures. It can all seem so hopeless, and we, as individuals, often feel small and powerless.

So how *can* we heal?

I believe that the first step is to collectively wake up and *accept what is*—because denial or resistance only blocks the progress we need to make. The next step is to become alert for toxic thought patterns, both individually and collectively projected by the media. These include blaming, demonizing, and obsessing over gloomy projections. Such thought patterns only serve to antagonize or depress people.

Instead, we must focus on new thoughts, new solutions, and positive visions of the future. Remember: positive thoughts and beliefs can literally enable the creation of the futures we want. Just like those who were able to survive the concentration camps, we can change our thoughts—in essence, heal our collective Mental Body—which will literally imbue us with the will to survive and take the actions that can yield what writer Charles Eisenstein calls, "The more beautiful world our hearts know is possible."[8]

The town Steve and I moved to in South Carolina is a case in point. It emerged from a dismal period of decline during the 60s and 70s and is now thriving, growing, and is palpably happier than the San Francisco Bay Area we left. The city's leaders created in a vision in the late 70s and used their will and effort—and I believe the city's collective Causal Body too—to make it happen. We saw and felt this energy the first day we arrived, and we are so glad we followed those energetic vibes!

COLLECTIVE HEALING AT THE CAUSAL LEVEL

As I have stressed throughout this book, the higher up we go in our healing activities, the more effective our efforts can be. By engaging with the hidden part of us that dwells on the causal level, we are able to heal on every level. And when we do so collectively, our potential power is even greater.

Do you doubt this is possible? Consider experiments conducted to test whether group meditations could lessen regional crime. One of the earliest such efforts was conducted during the summer of 1993 and enlisted 4000 practitioners of transcendental meditation to focus on lessening crime in Washington, D.C. The experiment was overseen by independent scientists. The data derived from police and FBI reports during the test period were statistically analyzed, taking into account all possible contributing factors. The results showed that homicides, rapes, and assaults dropped significantly during the test period with no other possible explanation, with the greatest drop occurring when the greatest number of meditators participated.[9]

Since that time, there have been many such collective meditation efforts, including an increasing number occurring over the internet. These global internet meditations are being organized to accomplish things like physical healing, alleviating violence and war, and creating peaceful and positive outcomes for our planet. Two organizations that regularly engage in these kinds of activities are Unify[10] and Lynn McTaggart's organization.[11]

To sum it up, each of us is inextricably part of a collective, no matter how isolated we may feel. How you feel each day—physically, energetically, emotionally, mentally, and spiritually—is affected by others, and you, too, have power to affect your environment and make a difference. Remember, as well, that our joint creations aren't just going on in the outer physical world. Something is always brewing in the interacting energies of the etheric level and within the giant emotional astral stew we participate in. Similarly, our individual wills are contributing to and affected by the mental energies of the collective. Finally, each of us is a single creator within a much larger creative causal organism—the Causal Body of humanity.

What will we create together?

CHAPTER 20

ン

WE ARE ONE

By now, at the end of this journey, it may be obvious: not only are we individuals, and not only are we participating in interactions at every level of our being, but ultimately, we are all part of *one* being. In other words, *we are one*—and not just one with the rest of humanity. We are one with the Earth and everything on it. We may even be one with our solar system, galaxy, and the universe! But for now, let's consider the implications of our oneness with Gaia—a name that has been used for the collective being that is all of Earth and everything on and within it.

Gaia has many levels, just as we all do, from the physical to the causal. On the physical level, he/she/it (let's use she) has organ systems and cells. Gaia's waters and even our human road systems might be her circulatory system. The atmosphere could be her respiratory system, and the giant plant and animal communications networks—including our own internet—might be her neurological system.

Then there are all the creeping, crawling, running, and swimming creatures on Gaia, including us humans. Are we her cells, much like the red blood cells travelling within us? Or are we more like the bacteria, viruses, and fungi within Gaia's microbiome? And just like the components of our own microbiome, humanity might be beneficial to Gaia or become harmful and lead to disease.

What about Gaia's Etheric Body? It includes the Etheric Bodies of all living beings on Earth, just as the Etheric Bodies of the bacteria and viruses within our own microbiome are part of our Etheric Body. Then there are the various etheric channels and points within Gaia's Etheric Body, analogous to our meridians and chakras. Some spiritual traditions talk about energetic *ley lines* that crisscross Earth, with certain locations— called *vortices*—functioning as special points of energy interchange. Are these Gaia's acupuncture points?

My husband Steve and I once visited Sedona, Arizona, which many people view as one such location. Others include Stonehenge, the pyramids, and Macchu Picchu. That is why human cultures have built spiritual structures there. Sedona is certainly a beautiful and mysterious locale, with its otherworldly red hills set amidst the Arizona desert. While we were there, we went on a "vortex tour" that took us to special spots in order to meditate. Amazingly, Steve "received" the entire plot for one of his novels during one of these meditations. Could vortices truly be places where energies enter and exit Gaia's Etheric Body?

Now let's consider Gaia's emotional Astral Body, which includes all of our own Astral Bodies. How does Gaia truly feel, deep down inside? Don't forget that her Astral Body holds the collective memory of Earth's entire history, going all the way back to her birth out of stellar dust. The volcanic eruptions, the bombardment by meteors, the various extinctions and glacial periods, and the history of all of humanity's travails, wars, and triumphs—it's all there. And of course, Gaia's Astral Body is psychic too. Perhaps she even communicates with the Astral Bodies of other planets in our solar system and the sun. Maybe that's why astrology can sometimes be an effective predictor of our own inner states.

Next comes Gaia's Mental Body. What is her mental purpose and will? Where are we as a planet going? Do we dare give up when the chips are down, when all is looking bleak? Shouldn't we, as a collective, focus on a better future, with a determined will—pushing through no matter what happens? And because our own Causal Body is a fragment of

Gaia's, that means we each need to wake up and envision the future we want. Then, when we unite, we can create whatever it is we focus on and believe. In other words, now, more than ever, it's imperative that we work together to heal at every level of our collective being and get in sync with what is and what we want.

So what will it take?

If we take an allopathic mindset, we will conduct various scientific tests, analyze the data, make a diagnosis, and apply a "pharmaceutical" or some "surgical" cut-and-paste solution. That's what we've been doing so far in order to solve Gaia's physical problems. Just like conventional medical doctors, today's ecological scientists study Gaia's symptoms and attempt to find answers. Unfortunately, they are sometimes misguided and create more problems down the line.

Take for example, drastic ecological "solutions"—like spraying particles into the atmosphere in order to create cloud cover. What consequences could this practice yield down the line? And is it really all about CO_2 numbers that must be reduced at all costs—even if it means collapsing our food supplies and losing our freedom? Indeed, some now believe that such efforts are being pushed by forces whose true motivations are much more nefarious.

And let's not forget our global societal and emotional problems. Short-term "band-aid" solutions are increasingly insufficient and sometimes dangerous if they involve imposing extreme levels of control over humanity. Are such solutions analogous to using chemotherapy for cancer, which sometimes ends up killing the patient rather than curing them? Or are they much like the pervasive belief in taking statins to reduce cholesterol numbers, which many now believe are actually bogus indicators of heart disease?

Sadly, even if they are well-intentioned, many proposed solutions for Gaia may be foolhardy and short-sighted. They tend to suppress symptoms, a strategy that alternative modalities like homeopathy tell us usually leads to deeper systemic problems down the line. Instead, we need to address problems at their root and utilize the natural healing powers of Gaia to our advantage. Authors like the brilliant Charles Eisenstein, in his book *Climate: A New Story*,[1] think so. Eisenstein suggests a more bottom-up approach. Just like cleaning up our diet is a better solution than popping another pill, healing the various ecosystems of Gaia and reducing pollution will enable her to correct and heal herself most beneficently. More nuanced solutions to Gaia's etheric, emotional, and mental wounds could also be found. In other words, holistic perspectives on human health and healing could provide us with clues and solutions for Gaia too.

Despite the seemingly dismal state of today's world, it's important to realize that there is definitely hope. *All is not lost.* We have our healing tools. Indeed, perhaps what we are currently experiencing is a part of some mysterious, synchronistic healing process. We need to face what's going on, not simply patch it over and run away from it with more distractions. We need to get in synchrony with *what is*.

Maybe that's why so many skeletons have been coming out of the closet lately. Despite their downsides, perhaps smartphones and the internet are letting us see various truths up close and making them harder to patch over and ignore. Could our growing awareness of surveillance, censorship, and increasing environmental degradation lead to a healing transformation for Gaia and humanity? A leap into an entirely new chapter for us? More and more, people are coming together to heal our global wounds and wake up to the structural powers that have enslaved our bodies, emotions, and minds. We may be at a tipping point, a pivotal and chaotic time of great positive potential. *And it's at times like these that we most need to focus, individually and collectively, on the future we **want**, rather than on the future we fear.*

Move Forward into Healing

This book's goal has been to impart a greater awareness of what we truly are. Using this information, each of us can begin to work on our own personal healing and transformation and then connect with others and the rest of Gaia to heal as a collective. I'll conclude now with eight key takeaways to keep in mind as you embark on this journey.

1. We are composed of many levels of being: physical, etheric, astral, mental, and causal.

2. Within each level, there is an interconnected and interacting collective in which we participate and that we are affected by. This collective includes not only all of humanity, but the entirety of Gaia—the animals, plants, waters, mountains, soil, minerals, and atmosphere.

3. All levels are interconnected with one another and affect each other.

4. When a change occurs at any level, it can propagate within that level *and* to all other levels. The higher up the level, the more inherently powerful the effects of a change can be.

5. Changes within the collective have more influence than changes within an individual.

6. A very small change is capable of creating a big effect, especially if it occurs at the right time, right place, and in the right way. This explains how an energetic dose of a perfectly-chosen homeopathic remedy can create huge effects. It also explains how a simple Sedona release can create significant emotional healing, and how a little bit of loving connection can dispel intense fear and anger.

7. Synchronicity (resonance between like-meaning energies) is a fundamental mechanism that creates effects at all levels and can serve as a method of communication between levels.

8. Because of mechanisms like synchronicity, what we believe, intend, feel, and think about (whether consciously or unconsciously) can have a dramatic effect upon our experiences at every level.

These eight essential points have at least four implications.

First, *we need to work on our beliefs, thoughts, and emotions.* That means blocking and, ideally, removing nocebos. It also means healing the habit of obsessing over dire future scenarios (which only programs the astral collective to manifest them) and, instead, focusing on *positive* visions and actions. For example, we need to create entertainments that illustrate a positive future for humanity, not an apocalypse.

Second, *we need to do this on all levels.* Change is not only required on the physical level. We must work on the etheric, astral, mental, and causal levels too. Each person will naturally gravitate to the level and activities that suit them personally. Some people may become activists on the physical level. Others will work on cleaning up the etheric environment or on helping people to release emotionally, become clearer mentally, or to create and manifest.

Third, *we must all be part of the effort.* The greater the collective, the greater the effect.

Finally, *we must protect who we are as natural human beings. If our access to any of the levels of our being is cut off, much of what I've described in this book will become impossible.* Not only can disruptions in the electromagnetic spectrum affect the etheric milieu in which we live and thus our Etheric Bodies, but I believe that following the "transhumanist" agenda and altering the nature of our Physical Body in fundamental ways will compromise who we are as human beings and disempower us. We cannot allow this to happen!

In other words, *it's time to align at every level—both within ourselves and with all of the milieus we exist within.* **It's time for us to learn to live in synchrony.**

In the end, we are part of one giant collective. As a result, we can't help but be affected by and, in some sense, "synchronize" with *what is*. The question is, will we be part of a grand harmonious symphony? Or will we relegate ourselves to a sorrowful, difficult, and unhealthy cacophony? It's finally time for each of us to "get in tune" and then sync up with others to create a more joyful and healthy Gaia.

NOTES AND RESOURCES

Chapter 1. It's All About Vibration

1. D. Radin. *Entangled Minds: Extrasensory Experiences in a Quantum Reality*. Paraview (2006).

    And L. McTaggart. *The Intention Experiment: Using Your Thoughts to Change Your Life and the World*. Free Press, pp. 56-61 (2007).

2. L. McTaggart. *The Intention Experiment: Using Your Thoughts to Change Your Life and the World*. Free Press, p.179-181(2007).

Chapter 3. Open and Expand Your View

1. D. Radin. *The Conscious Universe: The Scientific Truth of Psychic Phenomena*. HarperOne (2009).

    D. Radin. *Real Magic: Ancient Wisdom, Modern Science, and a Guide to the Secret Power of the Universe*. Harmony (2018).

    D. Radin. *Entangled Minds: Extrasensory Experiences in a Quantum Reality*. Paraview (2006).

2. L. McTaggart. *The Intention Experiment: Using Your Thoughts to Change Your Life and the World*. New York: Free Press, p.179-181(2007).

3. R. Targ. *Third Eye Spies: Learn Remote Viewing from the Masters*. New Page books (2023).

4. R. Sheldrake. *The Presence of the Past: Morphic Resonance and the Habits of Nature*. Park Street Press (1988).

    R. Sheldrake. *Seven Experiments That Could Change the World*. Park Street Press (1995).

5. K. Wilber. *A Brief History of Everything*. Shambhala (2000).

Chapter 4. The Box

1. www.psychologytoday.com/us/blog/going-beyond-intelligence/
   201711/why-parents-really-need-put-down-their-phones
2. www.scientificamerican.com/article/neuroscience-reveals-the-
   secrets-of-meditation-s-benefits/
3. T. Brach. *Radical Compassion: Learning to Love Yourself and Your World
   with the Practice of RAIN.* Penguin Life (2020).
4. www.bronnikovcenter.net

Chapter 5. Who Are We? What Are We?

1. A. Lansky. *Active Consciousness: Awakening the Power Within.*
   R.L.Ranch Press (2011).

Chapter 5 Resources

Steiner: R. Steiner. *Anthroposophy and the Inner Life: An Esoteric
Introduction.* Rudolf Steiner Press (1931).

Gurdjieff: P.D. Ouspensky. *In Search of the Miraculous: The Teachings of
G.I. Gurdjieff.* Harcourt, Inc. (1949).

Barbara Brennan: B.A. Brennan. *Hands of Light: A Guide to Healing
Through the Human Energy Field.* Bantam Books (1987).

Huna: C. Berney. *Fundamentals of Hawaiian Mysticism.* Crossing Press
(2000).

N. Veary. *Change We Must: My Spiritual Journey.* Water Margin Press
(1989).

M. Freedom Long. *The Secret Science At Work.* DeVorss & Company
(1953).

IAC: www.iacworld.org

M. Newton. *Journey of Souls.* Llewellyn Publications (1994).

A Course in Miracles. Foundation for Inner Peace (1975).

Lansky, Amy L. *Impossible Cure: The Promise of Homeopathy.* R.L.Ranch
Press (2003).

Chapter 6. Beyond the Physical and Etheric: The Higher Energy Bodies

1. C. Berney. *Fundamentals of Hawaiian Mysticism*. Crossing Press (2000).
   N. Veary. *Change We Must: My Spiritual Journey*. Water Margin Press (1989).
   M. Freedom Long. *The Secret Science At Work*. DeVorss & Company (1953).
2. www.iacworld.org
3. M. Newton. *Journey of Souls*. Llewellyn Publications (1994).
4. atransc.org/about-aaevp/   psychicscience.org/evp
   vimeo.com/101171248
5. nsac.org
6. H. Wesselman. *Spiritwalker: Messages from the Future*. Bantam (1996).

Chapter 8. I Think *and* I Am

1. J. Sarno. *Mind Over Back Pain*. Berkley (1999). J. Sarno. *The Divided Mind: The Epidemic of Mindbody Disorders*. HarperCollins (2007).
2. N. Goddard. *Neville Goddard: The Complete Reader: Imagining Creates Reality*. Audio Enlightenment (2013).
3. A. Lansky. *Active Consciousness: Awakening the Power Within*. R.L.Ranch Press (2011).
4. C.G. Jung. *Memories, Dreams, and Reflections*. Vintage (1989).

Chapter 9. Opening the Door of Creation

1. M. Freedom Long. *The Secret Science At Work*. DeVorss & Company (1953).
2. F.S. Shinn. *The Game of Life & How to Play It*. Sound Wisdom (2019).
3. N. Goddard. *Neville Goddard: The Complete Reader: Imagining Creates Reality*. Audio Enlightenment (2013).
4. T. Silver. *Outrageous Openness: Letting the Divine Take the Lead*. Atria Paperback (2016).

Chapter 11. A Greater Cosmology

1. T. Halliwell. *Summer with the Leprechauns*. Tanis Helliwell Corporation (2011).
2. P. Hawken. *The Magic of Findhorn*. Bantam Books (1976).
3. M.S. Wright. *Behaving As If the God in All Life Mattered*. Perelandra (1997).
4. *Nosso Lar (Astral City)*.
    en.wikipedia.org/wiki/Astral_City:_A_Spiritual_Journey.
5. J. Roberts. *Seth Speaks: The Eternal Validity of the Soul*. Amber-Allen Publications, New World Library (1994).

Chapter 12. The Purpose of Life

1. N. Goddard. *Neville Goddard: The Complete Reader: Imagining Creates Reality*. Audio Enlightenment (2013).
2. M. Dooley. *Life on Earth*. Hay House Inc. (2016).
3. A. Moorjani. *Dying to Be Me*. Hay House LLC (2022).
    A. Moorjani. *What If This Is Heaven?* Hay House LLC (2017).

Chapter 13. Healing From the Outside In

1. C. Berney. *Fundamentals of Hawaiian Mysticism*. Crossing Press (2000).
2. www.resperate.com

Chapter 13 Resources

Hypnotherarpy: A. Alamillo. *The Dark Side of the Mind*. (2015).
Cognitive Behavioral Therapy for Insomnia: SHUT-I (myshuti.com).
Mind Over Body: J. Dispenza. *You Are the Placebo*. Hay House LLC (2015).
    H. Dwoskin. *The Sedona Method*. Sedona Press (2003).
    J. Sarno. *Mind Over Back Pain*. Berkley (1999).
    J. Sarno. *The Divided Mind: The Epidemic of Mindbody Disorders*. HarperCollins (2007).
Logosynthesis: *www.logosynthesis.net*

L. Hay. *You Can Heal Your Life.* Hay House LLC (1984).

Trauma: TRE: traumaprevention.com

K. Neff. *Self-Compassion: The Proven Power of Being Kind to Yourself.* William Morrow (2015).

T. Brach. *Radical Acceptance.* Bantam (2004).

Manifestation: N. Goddard. *Neville Goddard: The Complete Reader: Imagining Creates Reality.* Audio Enlightenment (2013).

T. Silver. *Outrageous Openness: Letting the Divine Take the Lead.* Atria Paperback (2016). E. Holmes.

The Science of Mind. Tarcher Perigee (2010).

T. Troward. *Thomas Troward Complete Collection.* (2019).

Spiritual: M. Singer. *The Untethered Soul.* New Harbinger/Noetic Books (2007).

M. Singer. *The Surrender Experiment.* Harmony (2015). A.C. Bailey and C.B. Marlowe.

The Trust Frequency. Cameron/Baxter Books (2018).

M. Dooley. *Life on Earth.* Hay House Inc. (2016).

A. Moorjani. *Dying to Be Me.* Hay House LLC (2022).

A. Moorjani. *What If This Is Heaven?* Hay House LLC (2017).

A Course in Miracles. Foundation for Inner Peace (1975).

Chapter 14. We Are Physical Beings

1. S. Lupkin. *One-Third of New Drugs Had Safety Problems After FDA Approval.* NPR (May 9, 2017).
2. www.viome.com
3. D. Chopra. *Perfect Health.* Harmony (2007).
4. gokhalemethod.com
5. alexandertechnique.com
   F. M. Alexander. *The Use of the Self.* Spring (2019).
6. aomtinfo.org/myofunctional-therapy/
   iaom.com
7. E. Gokhale. *8 Steps to a Pain-Free Back.* Pendo Press (2008).

8. www.zonetechniquesite.com/zone-technique

Chapter 15. We Are Beings Governed by Energy and Vibration

1. A. Lansky. *Impossible Cure: The Promise of Homeopathy.* RL Ranch Press (2003).
2. homeopathychoice.org
3. L. Montagnier, et al. *Electromagnetic Signals Are Produced by Aqueous Nanostructures Derived from Bacterial DNA Sequences.* Interdiscip Sci Comput Life Sci (2009). www.huffpost.com/entry/luc-montagnier-homeopathy-taken-seriously_b_814619
4. J. Aissa, et al. "Transatlantic Transfer of Digitized Antigen Signal by Telephone Link." *Journal of Allergy and Clinical Immunology,* 99:S175 (1997). homeopathic.com/science-friction-homeopathy-vs-the-debunkers/
5. B.A. Brennan. *Hands of Light: A Guide to Healing Through the Human Energy Field.* Bantam Books (1987).
6. R. Gordon. *Quantum-Touch: The Power to Heal.* North Atlantic Books (2006).
7. D. Wardell, S. Kagel, and L. Anselme. *Healing Touch: Enhancing Life through Energy Therapy.* (2014).
8. D. Stein. *Essential Reiki: A Complete Guide to an Ancient Healing Art.* Crossing Press (1995).
9. www.sensiblehealth.com/Y-Dan.xhtml
   en.wikipedia.org/wiki/Qigong
10. C. Swanson. *Life Force, The Scientific Basis.* Poseidia Press (2011).
11. hemi-sync.com
    www.monroeinstitute.org
12. M. Emoto. *The Hidden Messages in Water.* Simon & Schuster (2005).
13. E.D. McKusick. *Electric Body, Electric Health.* Essentials (2021).
    E.D. McKusick. *Tuning the Human Biofield: Healing with Vibrational Sound.* Healing Arts Press (2021).
14. emfacademy.com/shungite-complete-honest-guide/

S.P. Kurotchenko, etal. *Shielding Effect of Mineral Schungite During Electromagnetic Irradiation of Rats.* Bull Exp Biol Med. November; 136(5):458-9 (2003).

15. L.K. Chuen. *Feng Shui Handbook.* Henry Holt (1996).
16. I. Karim. *BioGeometry Signatures: Harmonizing the Body's Subtle Energy Exchange with the Environment.* (2016).

Chapter 16. We Are Emotional Psychic Beings

1. P.D. Ouspensky. *In Search of the Miraculous: The Teachings of G.I. Gurdjieff.* Harcourt, Inc. (1949).
2. E. Langer. *Counterclockwise.* Hodder Paperback (2010).
3. J. Dispenza. *You Are the Placebo.* Hay House LLC (2015).
4. J. Sarno. *Mind Over Back Pain.* Berkley (1999).
   J. Sarno. *The Divided Mind: The Epidemic of Mindbody Disorders.* HarperCollins (2007).
5. A. Alamillo. *The Dark Side of the Mind.* (2015).
6. L. Hay. *You Can Heal Your Life.* Hay House LLC (1984).
7. E. Holmes. *The Science of Mind.* Tarcher Perigee (2010).
8. Centers for Spiritual Living: csl.org
9. K. Neff. *Self-Compassion: The Proven Power of Being Kind to Yourself.* William Morrow (2015).
10. H. Dwoskin. *The Sedona Method.* Sedona Press (2003). www.sedona.com
11. M. Singer. *The Surrender Experiment.* Harmony (2015).
12. www.coretransformation.org
13. J. Manne. *Family Constellations.* North Atlantic Books (2009).
14. G. Craig. *The EFT Manual.* Energy Psychology Press (2008). eftinternational.org
15. H. Grayson. *Your Power to Heal: Resolving Psychological Barriers to Your Physical Health.* Sounds True (2017).
16. F. Shapiro. *Eye Movement Desensitization and Reprocessing (EMDR) Therapy.* The Guilford Press (2017). www.emdr.com

17. TRE: traumaprevention.com
18. www.goodtherapy.org/learn-about-therapy/types/breathwork
19. ecstaticdance.org
20. G. Hancock. *Visionary (The Definitive Edition of Supernatural)*. New Page Books (2022).

Chapter 17. We Are Willful, Thinking, Meaning-full Beings

1. G. Sherman. *Perceptual Integration: The Mechanics of Awakening*. Inner Harmonics Press (2013)
2. V. Frankl. *Man's Search for Meaning*. Beacon Press (2006).
3. B. Katie. *Loving What Is*. Harmony (2021).
4. Logosynthesis: www.logosynthesis.net
5. M. Desmet. *The Psychology of Totalitarianism*. Chelsea Green Publishing (2022).

Chapter 18. We Are Creators

1. A. Lansky. *Active Consciousness: Awakening the Power Within*. R.L.Ranch Press, pp.127-130 (2011).
2. E.R. Gruber. "Conformance Behavior Involving Animal and Human Subject." *European Journal of Parapsychology*, 3(1), pp. 36-50 (2007). Also see discussion in L. McTaggart. *The Intention Experiment: Using Your Thoughts to Change Your Life and the World*. New York: Free Press, p.166-174 (2007).
3. E. Hicks and J. Hicks. *The Amazing Power of Deliberate Intent*. Hay House (2006).
4. T. Silver. *Outrageous Openness: Letting the Divine Take the Lead*. Atria Paperback (2016).
5. www.oprahdaily.com/life/a30244004/how-to-manifest-anything/
6. D. Chopra. *Synchrodestiny*. Rider (2003).
7. H. Dwoskin. *The Sedona Method*. Sedona Press (2003).
8. J. Dispenza. *You Are the Placebo*. Hay House LLC (2015).
9. W. Dyer. *Wishes Fulfilled: Mastering the Art of Manifesting*. Hay House

(2013).

10. L. Hay. *You Can Heal Your Life*. Hay House (1984).

11. R. Byrne. *The Secret*. Simon and Schuster (1994).

12. J. Roberts. *Seth Speaks: The Eternal Validity of the Soul*. Amber-Allen Publications, New World Library (1994).

13. *A Course in Miracles*. Foundation for Inner Peace (1975).

14. S. Roman. *Living With Joy*. HJ Kramer (2011).
    S. Roman. *Personal Power Through Awareness*. HJ Kramer (2019).
    S. Roman. *Spiritual Growth*. HJ Kramer (1992).

15. www.dalecarnegie.com

16. www.naphill.org

17. N. Goddard. *Neville Goddard: The Complete Reader: Imagining Creates Reality*. Audio Enlightenment (2013).

18. F.S. Shinn. *The Game of Life & How to Play It*. Sound Wisdom (2019).

19. J. Allen. *As A Man Thinketh*. Reader's Library Classics (2022).

20. www.pealefoundation.org

21. T. Troward. *Thomas Troward Complete Collection*. (2019).

22. E. Holmes. *The Science of Mind*. Tarcher Perigee (2010).

23. Centers for Spiritual Living: csl.org

24. C. Berney. *Fundamentals of Hawaiian Mysticism*. Crossing Press (2000).
    N. Veary. *Change We Must: My Spiritual Journey*. Water Margin Press (1989).
    M. Freedom Long. *The Secret Science At Work*. DeVorss & Company (1953).

25. C.G. Jung. *Memories, Dreams, and Reflections*. Vintage (1989).

26. R. Steiner. *Anthroposophy and the Inner Life: An Esoteric Introduction*. Rudolf Steiner Press (1931).

27. P.D. Ouspensky. *In Search of the Miraculous: The Teachings of G.I. Gurdjieff*. Harcourt, Inc. (1949).

28. emersoncentral.com

29. www.thoreau-online.org

30. nsac.org
31. www.christianscience.com/what-is-christian-science/mary-baker-eddy
32. swedenborg.com
33. A.C. Bailey and C.B. Marlowe. *The Trust Frequency.* Cameron/Baxter Books (2018).
34. M. Singer. *The Surrender Experiment.* Harmony (2015).

Chapter 19. You Are Not Alone

1. D. Radin. "Exploring Relationships Between Random Physical Events and Mass Human Intention: Asking for Whom the Bell Tolls." *Journal of Scientific Exploration.* 16(4), pp. 533-547 (2002).
2. www.biggestlittlefarmmovie.com
3. pubmed.ncbi.nlm.nih.gov/20674839/
   G. Bracho, et al. "Large-scale application of highly-diluted bacteria for Leptospirosis epidemic control." *Homeopathy.* July; 99(3):156-166 (2010).
4. D. Castro and G. Nogueria, "Use of the Nosode Meningococcinum As a Preventative Against Meningitis," *Journal of the American Institute of Homeopathy,* 68:211-219 (1975).
5. www.homeopathyforhealthinafrica.org arhf.nl/en/home
6. T. Hubl. *Healing Collective Trauma.* Sounds True Adult (2023).
7. M. Desmet. *The Psychology of Totalitarianism.* Chelsea Green Publishing (2022).
8. C. Eisenstein. *The More Beautiful World Our Hearts Know Is Possible.* North Atlantic Books (2013).
9. J.S. Hagelin, et al. "Effects of Group Practice of the Transcendental Meditation Program on Preventing Violent Crime in Washington, DC: Results of the National Demonstration Project, June–July 1993." *Social Indicators Research,* 47: 153–201 (1999).

D.W. Orme-Johnson, et al. "Preventing Terrorism and International Conflict: Effects of Large Assemblies of Participants in the Transcendental Meditation and TM-Sidhi Programs." *Journal of Offender Rehabilitation*, 36: 283–302 (2003).
10. www.unify.org
11. lynnemctaggart.com

Chapter 20. Ultimately, We Are One
1. C. Eisenstein. *Climate: A New Story*. North Atlantic Books (2018).

BIBLIOGRAPHY

A Course in Miracles. Foundation for Inner Peace (1975).

Aissa, J. et al. "Transatlantic Transfer of Digitized Antigen Signal by Telephone Link." *Journal of Allergy and Clinical Immunology*, 99:S175 (1997).

Alamillo, A. *The Dark Side of the Mind*. Alba Alamillo (2015).

Alexander, F.M. *The Use of the Self*. Spring (2019).

Allen, J. *As A Man Thinketh*. Reader's Library Classics (2022).

Andreas, C. and T, Andreas. *Core Transformation: Reaching the Wellspring*. Real People Press (2015).

Bailey, A.C. and C.B. Marlowe. *The Trust Frequency*. Cameron/Baxter Books (2018).

Berceli, D. *Trauma Releasing Exercises (TRE): A Revolutionary New Method for Stress/Trauma Recovery*. BookSurge Publishing (2005).

Berney, C. *Fundamentals of Hawaiian Mysticism*. Crossing Press (2000).

Brach, G. et al. "Large-scale application of highly-diluted bacteria for Leptospirosis epidemic control." *Homeopathy*. July; 99(3):156–166 (2010).

Brach, T. *Radical Acceptance*. Bantam (2004).

Brach, T. *Radical Compassion: Learning to Love Yourself and Your World with the Practice of RAIN*. Penguin Life (2020).

Brennan, B.A. *Hands of Light: A Guide to Healing Through the Human Energy Field*. Bantam Books (1987).

Byrne, R. *The Secret*. Simon and Schuster (1994).

Carnegie, D. *How to Stop Worrying and Start Living*. Gallery Books (2004).

Carnegie, D. *How to Win Friends and Influence People*. Pocket Books (1998).

Castro, D. and G. Nogueria, "Use of the Nosode Meningococcinum as a Preventative Against Meningitis," *Journal of the American Institute of Homeopathy*, 68:211–219 (1975).

Chopra. D. *Perfect Health*. Harmony (2007).

Chopra, D. *Synchrodestiny*. Rider (2003).

Chuen, L.K. *Feng Shui Handbook*. Henry Holt (1996).

Craig, G. *The EFT Manual*. Energy Psychology Press (2008).

Desmet, M. *The Psychology of Totalitarianism*. Chelsea Green Publishing (2022).

Dispenza, J. *You Are the Placebo*. Hay House LLC (2015).

Dooley, M. *Life on Earth*. Hay House Inc. (2016).

Dwoskin, H. *The Sedona Method*. Sedona Press (2003).

Dyer, W. *Wishes Fulfilled: Mastering the Art of Manifesting*. Hay House (2013).

Eisenstein, C. *Climate: A New Story*. North Atlantic Books (2018).

Eisenstein, C. *The More Beautiful World Our Hearts Know Is Possible*. North Atlantic Books (2013).

Emerson, R.W. *The Essential Writings of Ralph Waldo Emerson*. Modern Library (2000).

Emoto, M. *The Hidden Messages in Water*. Simon & Schuster (2005).

Frankl, V. *Man's Search for Meaning*. Beacon Press (2006).

Goddard, N. *Neville Goddard: The Complete Reader: Imagining Creates Reality*. Audio Enlightenment (2013).

Gokhale, E. *8 Steps to a Pain-Free Back*. Pendo Press (2008).

Gordon, R. *Quantum-Touch: The Power to Heal*. North Atlantic Books (2006).

Grayson, H. *Your Power to Heal: Resolving Psychological Barriers to Your Physical Health*. Sounds True (2017).

Gruber, E.R. "Conformance Behavior Involving Animal and Human Subject." *European Journal of Parapsychology*, 3(1), pp. 36-50 (2007).

Hagelin, J.S. et al. "Effects of Group Practice of the Transcendental Meditation Program on Preventing Violent Crime in Washington, DC: Results of the National Demonstration Project, June–July 1993." *Social Indicators Research*, 47: 153–201 (1999).

Halliwell. *Summer with the Leprechauns,* T. Tanis Helliwell Corporation (2011).

Hancock, G. *Visionary (The Definitive Edition of Supernatural).* New Page Books (2022).

Hawken, P. *The Magic of Findhorn.* Bantam Books (1976).

Hay, L. *You Can Heal Your Life.* Hay House LLC (1984).

Hicks, E. and J. Hicks. *The Amazing Power of Deliberate Intent.* Hay House (2006).

Holmes, E. *The Science of Mind.* Tarcher Perigee (2010).

Hubl, T. *Healing Collective Trauma.* Sounds True Adult (2023).

Jung, C.G. *Memories, Dreams, and Reflections.* Vintage (1989).

Karim, I. *BioGeometry Signatures: Harmonizing the Body's Subtle Energy Exchange with the Environment.* Createspace (2016).

Katie, B. *Loving What Is.* Harmony (2021).

Kurotchenko, S.P. et al. *Shielding Effect of Mineral Schungite During Electromagnetic Irradiation of Rats.* Bull Exp Biol Med. November; 136(5):458-9 (2003).

Lammers, W. *Discover Logosynthesis: The Power of Words in Healing and Development* (2020).

Langer, E. *Counterclockwise.* Hodder Paperback (2010).

Lansky, A. *Active Consciousness: Awakening the Power Within.* R.L.Ranch Press (2011).

Lansky, A. *Impossible Cure: The Promise of Homeopathy.* R.L.Ranch Press (2003).

Long, M. Freedom. *The Secret Science at Work.* DeVorss & Company (1953).

Manne, J. *Family Constellations.* North Atlantic Books (2009).

McKusick, E.D. *Electric Body, Electric Health.* Essentials (2021).

McKusick, E.D. *Tuning the Human Biofield: Healing with Vibrational Sound.* Healing Arts Press (2021).

McTaggart, L. *The Intention Experiment: Using Your Thoughts to Change Your Life and the World.* Free Press (2007).

Montagnier, L. et al. *Electromagnetic Signals Are Produced by Aqueous Nanostructures Derived from Bacterial DNA Sequences.* Interdiscip Sci Comput Life Sci (2009).

Moorjani, A. *Dying to Be Me.* Hay House (2022).

Moorjani, A. *What If This Is Heaven?* Hay House (2017).

Neff, K. *Self-Compassion: The Proven Power of Being Kind to Yourself.* William Morrow (2015).

Newton, M. *Journey of Souls.* Llewellyn Publications (1994).

Nosso Lar (Astral City). en.wikipedia.org/wiki/Astral_City:_A_Spiritual_Journey

Orme-Johnson, D.W. et al. "Preventing Terrorism and International Conflict: Effects of Large Assemblies of Participants in the Transcendental Meditation and TM-Sidhi Programs." *Journal of Offender Rehabilitation*, 36: 283–302 (2003).

Ouspensky, P.D. *In Search of the Miraculous: The Teachings of G.I. Gurdjieff.* Harcourt, Inc. (1949).

Radin, D. *The Conscious Universe: The Scientific Truth of Psychic Phenomena.* HarperOne (2009).

Radin, D. *Entangled Minds: Extrasensory Experiences in a Quantum Reality.* Paraview (2006).

Radin, D. "Exploring Relationships Between Random Physical Events and Mass Human Intention: Asking for Whom the Bell Tolls." *Journal of Scientific Exploration.* 16(4), pp. 533-547 (2002).

Radin, D. *Real Magic: Ancient Wisdom, Modern Science, and a Guide to the Secret Power of the Universe.* Harmony (2018).

Roman, S. *Living With Joy.* HJ Kramer (2011).

Roman, S. *Personal Power Through Awareness.* HJ Kramer (2019).

Roman, S. *Spiritual Growth.* HJ Kramer (1992).

Roberts, J. *Seth Speaks: The Eternal Validity of the Soul.* Amber-Allen Publications, New World Library (1994).

Sarno, J. *Mind Over Back Pain.* Berkley (1999).

Sarno, J. *The Divided Mind: The Epidemic of Mindbody Disorders.* HarperCollins (2007).

Shapiro, F. *Eye Movement Desensitization and Reprocessing (EMDR) Therapy.* The Guilford Press (2017).

Sherman, G. *Perceptual Integration: The Mechanics of Awakening.* Inner Harmonics Press (2013)

Sheldrake, R. *The Presence of the Past: Morphic Resonance and the Habits of Nature.* Park Street Press (1988).

Sheldrake, R. *Seven Experiments That Could Change the World.* Park Street Press (1995).

Shinn, F.S. *The Game of Life & How to Play It.* Sound Wisdom (2019).

Silver, T. *Outrageous Openness: Letting the Divine Take the Lead.* Atria Paperback (2016).

Singer, M. *The Untethered Soul.* New Harbinger/Noetic Books (2007).

Singer, M. *The Surrender Experiment.* Harmony (2015).

Stein, D. *Essential Reiki: A Complete Guide to an Ancient Healing Art.* Crossing Press (1995).

Steiner, R. *Anthroposophy and the Inner Life: An Esoteric Introduction.* Rudolf Steiner Press (1931).

Swanson, C. *Life Force, The Scientific Basis.* Poseidia Press (2011).

Targ, R. *Third Eye Spies: Learn Remote Viewing from the Masters.* New Page books (2023).

Thoreau, H.D. *The Portable Thoreau.* Penguin Classics (2012).

Troward, T. *Thomas Troward Complete Collection* (2019).

Veary, N. *Change We Must: My Spiritual Journey.* Water Margin Press (1989).

Wardell, D., S. Kagel, and L. Anselme. *Healing Touch: Enhancing Life through Energy Therapy* (2014).

Wesselman, H. *Spiritwalker: Messages from the Future.* Bantam (1996).

Wilber, K. *A Brief History of Everything.* Shambhala (2000).

Wright, M.S. *Behaving As If the God in All Life Mattered.* Perelandra (1997).

Assorted Websites

Breathwork:
    www.goodtherapy.org/learn-about-therapy/types/breathwork

Chiropractic:
    www.zonetechniquesite.com/zone-technique

Core Transformation:
    www.coretransformation.org

Ecstatic Dance:
    ecstaticdance.org

EFT:
    eftinternational.org

EMDR:
    www.emdr.com

Homeopathy:
    homeopathycenter.org
    homeopathychoice.org
    www.huffpost.com/entry/luc-montagnier-homeopathy-taken-seriously_b_814619
    homeopathic.com/science-friction-homeopathy-vs-the-debunkers/pubmed.ncbi.nlm.nih.gov/20674839
    www.homeopathyforhealthinafrica.org/arhf.nl/en/home

IAC:
    www.iacworld.org

Insomnia:
    www.psychologytoday.com/us/blog/reading-between-the-headlines/201702/shuti-new-insomnia-treatment-the-internet

Logosynthesis:
    www.logosynthesis.net

Manifestation and Meditation:
    lynnemctaggart.com
    www.unify.org

www.scientificamerican.com/article/neuroscience-reveals-the-secrets-of-meditation-s-benefits/

New Thought:

Centers for Spiritual Living: csl.org

Christian Science: www.christianscience.com/what-is-christian-science/mary-baker-eddy

Dale Carnegie: www.dalecarnegie.com

Napoleon Hill: www.naphill.org

Norman Vincent Peale: www.pealefoundation.org

Posture:

gokhalemethod.com

alexandertechnique.com

aomtinfo.org/myofunctional-therapy

Psychic Powers and Phenomena:

www.bronnikovcenter.net

psychicscience.org/evp

Qi Gong:

www.sensiblehealth.com/Y-Dan.xhtml

en.wikipedia.org/wiki/Qigong

Regenerative Farming:

www.biggestlittlefarmmovie.com

Resperate:

www.resperate.com

Sedona Method:

www.sedona.com

Society and Family

www.psychologytoday.com/us/blog/going-beyond-intelligence/201711/why-parents-really-need-put-down-their-phones

Sound:

hemi-sync.com

www.monroeinstitute.org

Spiritualism and Afterlife Communication:

    nsac.org

    atransc.org/about-aaevp/

    vimeo.com/101171248

Swedenborgianism:

    swedenborg.com

Transcendentalism:

    emersoncentral.com

    www.thoreau-online.org

TRE:

    traumaprevention.com

Viome:

    www.viome.com

SELECTED INDEX

Abraham Hicks	253
Acupressure	167-168
Acupuncture	167-168
Allopathy	119-123
Applied Kinesiology	179
Astral Body	55-66, 180-217
Signs of dysfunction	182-185
Collective healing	267-270
Automatic Writing	201-204
Breathwork	213-215
Causal Body	55-57, 75-79, 237-255
Signs of dysfunction	246
Collective healing	273-274
Central Channel	51-52
Chiropractic	144-145
Collective Healing	256-274
Core Transformation	207-208
Crystals	176-178
Detoxification	133-136
Diet and Supplementation	123-130
Dispenza, Joe	251-252
Divas	93-95
Divination	201-204
Ecstatic Dance	213-215
EFT (Emotional Freedom Technique)	209-211
Elementals	93-95
EMDR (Eye Movement Desensitization and Reprocessing)	211-212
Energy Body Architecture	48, 92, 110-111

Etheric Body   49-53, 148-179
  Signs of dysfunction   151-154
  Collective healing   264-267
Family Constellation Therapy   208-209
Gaia   275-281
Geometric Healing   176-178
Goddard, Neville   250-251
Ha Ritual   81-85
Hands-On Healing   170-172
Herbalism   131-133
Higher Body   54
Homeopathy   157-166
Huna   56-57, 81-85, 249-250
Hypnotherapy   199-201
Journaling   201-204
Katie, Byron   229-231
Law of Attraction   239-242
Living in Synchrony   17-21, 279-281
Logosynthesis   232-233
Logotherapy   234-236
Lucid Dreams   64-66
Manifestation   241-245, 247-255
Massage   142-144
Meditation   40-41, 77
Mental Body   55-57, 71-75, 218-236
  Signs of dysfunction   225-226
  Collective healing   270-273
Microbiome   125-128
Mirror Work   204-205
Movement Therapy   142-144
New Thought   99, 242
Nocebo   189

Osteopathy	144-147
Out-of-Body Experiences	59-60, 64-66
Oversouls and Angels	95-96
Plant Medicine	215-217
Physical Body	48, 91-93, 114-147
Signs of dysfunction	116
Collective healing	260-264
Physical Therapy	137-138
Posture Therapy	139-142
Psychic Phenomena	26-28, 43, 58
Psychotherapy	197-198, 227-229
Reincarnation	55
Sarno, John and TMS	192-196
Science of Mind	253-254
Sedona Method	205-207
Self-compassion	204-205
Shamanism	215-217
Sound Therapy	174-176
Spiritualism	63, 243-244
Sweat Lodge	213-215
Synchronicity	25, 78, 220-221, 231-232, 242, 280
Tai Chi	172-173
TFT (Thought Field Therapy)	211
Traditional Chinese Medicine	166-169
Transhumanism	4, 33
TRE (Trauma Release Exercises)	212-213
Vibration	9-11
Will	221-223
Yoga	172-173

ABOUT THE AUTHOR

Even as a child growing up outside Buffalo, New York, Amy Lansky sensed that the world was a bit more mysterious than it appeared on the surface. After many years working as a research computer scientist in Silicon Valley, she decided to pursue her life passion—to uncover deeper truths hidden behind the veil of our consensual reality.

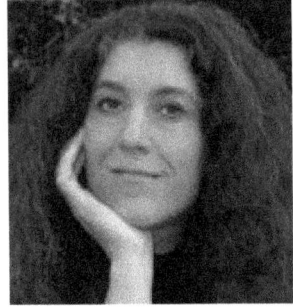

Lansky's first book, *Impossible Cure: The Promise of Homeopathy* (2003), explored an unconventional form of healing—homeopathy. It quickly became one of the best-selling introductory books on the subject and is still used as a patient education book and textbook all over the world. It is especially popular with families struggling with the autism epidemic. Her second book, *Active Consciousness: Awakening the Power Within* (2011), explored the mysterious realm of human consciousness.

In this, her third book, Lansky presents a model of the human energy bodies and their powerful role in determining our physical, emotional, and mental health. Based on years of exploration and experience with a wide variety of modalities, she provides healing guidance for us all—not just on an individual basis, but collectively too. At a time when global health systems are not only failing us, but actively undermining our healing abilities as natural human beings, her message is more timely than ever.

Lansky received her doctorate in computer science from Stanford University. After the miraculous homeopathic cure of her son's autism, she decided to leave the field to pursue her interest in homeopathic medicine. Later, in a search for health freedom during the COVID years, Lansky and her husband embarked upon a year-long voyage across America and now reside in the beautiful upstate area of South Carolina.

www.ingramcontent.com/pod-product-compliance
Lightning Source LLC
Chambersburg PA
CBHW031500270326
41930CB00006B/175